Health Informatics
(formerly Computers in Health Care)

Kathryn J. Hannah   Marion J. Ball
Series Editors

Springer
New York
Berlin
Heidelberg
Hong Kong
London
Milan
Paris
Tokyo

Health Informatics Series
(formerly Computers in Health Care)

Series Editors
Kathryn J. Hannah   Marion J. Ball

Dental Informatics
Integrating Technology into the Dental Environment
L.M. Abbey and J. Zimmerman

Ethics and Information Technology
A Case-Based Approach to a Health Care System in Transition
J.G. Anderson and K.W. Goodman

Aspects of the Computer-Based Patient Record
M.J. Ball and M.F. Collen

Performance Improvement Through Information Management
Health Care's Bridge to Success
M.J. Ball and J.V. Douglas

Strategies and Technologies for Healthcare Information
Theory into Practice
M.J. Ball, J.V. Douglas, and D.E. Garets

Nursing Informatics
Where Caring and Technology Meet, Third Edition
M.J. Ball, K.J. Hannah, S.K. Newbold, and J.V. Douglas

Healthcare Information Management Systems
A Practical Guide, Second Edition
M.J. Ball, D.W. Simborg, J.W. Albright, and J.V. Douglas

Clinical Decision Support Systems
Theory and Practice
E.S. Berner

Strategy and Architecture of Health Care Information Systems
M.K. Bourke

Information Networks for Community Health
P.F. Brennan, S.J. Schneider, and E. Tornquist

Informatics for the Clinical Laboratory
A Practical Guide
D.F. Cowan

Introduction to Clinical Informatics
P. Degoulet and M. Fieschi

(continued after index)

Rudi Van de Velde   Patrice Degoulet

Clinical Information Systems
A Component-Based Approach

With 125 Illustrations

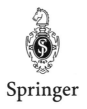

Springer

Rudi Van de Velde, Ph.D.
Professor at the Faculty of Medicine
Free University of Brussels
and
Department of Medical Informatics
AZ-VUB, University Hospital Brussels
101, Laarbeek Avenue
1090 Brussels, Belgium
rudi.vandevelde@az.vub.ac.be

Patrice Degoulet, M.D., Ph.D.
Professor at the Broussais Hôtel-Dieu
    Faculty of Medicine
University Pierre and Marie Curie
15, rue de l'Ecole de Médecine
75006 Paris, France
and
Department of Medical Informatics
HEGP, Georges Pompidou University Hospital
20, rue Leblanc
75015 Paris, France
patrice.degoulet@spim.jussieu.fr

Series Editors:

Kathryn J. Hannah, Ph.D., R.N.
Adjunct Professor, Department of
    Community Health Science
Faculty of Medicine
The University of Calgary
Calgary, Alberta T2N 4N1, Canada

Marion J. Ball, Ed.D.
Vice President, Clinical Solutions
Healthlink, Inc.
2 Hamill Road
Quadrangle 359 West
Baltimore, MD 21210
and
Adjunct Professor
The Johns Hopkins University
    School of Nursing
Baltimore, MD 21205, USA

Cover illustration: Cover art © Gary Nichols/Images.com.

Library of Congress Cataloging-in-Publication Data
Velde, Rudi Van de.
    Clinical information systems: a component-based approach/Rudi Van de Velde,
Patrice Degoulet.
        p.; cm. — (Health informatics)
    Includes bibliographical references and index.
    ISBN 0-387-95538-0 (alk. paper)
        1. Medicine—Data processing.   2. Hospital care—Data processing.   3. Information
storage and retrieval systems—Medicine.   4. Medical records—Data processing.
    I. Degoulet, Patrice.   II. Title.   III. Series.
        [DNLM: 1. Hospital Information Systems.   2. Community Networks.   3. Decision
Support Systems, Clinical.   4. Medical Records Systems, Computerized.   WX 26.5 V435c 2002]
    R858 .V445 2002
    610′.285—dc21   2002026668

ISBN 0-387-95538-0   Printed on acid-free paper.

Printed in the United States of America.

9 8 7 6 5 4 3 2 1   SPIN 10885436

Typesetting: Pages created by the authors using Adobe FrameMaker.

www.springer-ny.com

Springer-Verlag   New York Berlin Heidelberg
A member of BertelsmannSpringer Science+Business Media GmbH

To the memory of Jean-Raoul Scherrer

Series Preface

This series is directed to healthcare professionals who are leading the transformation of health care by using information and knowledge. Launched in 1988 as Computers in Health Care, the series offers a broad range of titles: some addressed to specific professions such as nursing, medicine, and health administration; others to special areas of practice such as trauma and radiology. Still other books in the series focus on interdisciplinary issues, such as the computer-based patient record, electronic health records, and networked healthcare systems.

Renamed Health Informatics in 1998 to reflect the rapid evolution in the discipline now known as health informatics, the series will continue to add titles that contribute to the evolution of the field. In the series, eminent experts, serving as editors or authors, offer their accounts of innovations in health informatics. Increasingly, these accounts go beyond hardware and software to address the role of information in influencing the transformation of healthcare delivery systems around the world. The series also increasingly focuses on "peopleware" and the organizational, behavioral, and societal changes that accompany the diffusion of information technology in health services environments.

These changes will shape health services in this new millennium. By making full and creative use of the technology to tame data and to transform information, health informatics will foster the development of the knowledge age in health care. As coeditors, we pledge to support our professional colleagues and the series readers as they share advances in the emerging and exciting field of health informatics.

Kathryn J. Hannah
Marion J. Ball

Preface

> *The reasonable man adapts himself to the world, the unreasonable man adapts the world to him. All progress depends on the unreasonable man.*
>
> —George Bernard Shaw

A hospital information system (HIS) may be defined as a computer system designed to ease the management of all the hospital's medical and administrative information, and to improve the quality of health care. The first HISs were developed in the mid-1960s in the United States and in a few European countries. HISs have followed the general evolutionary trends in computing systems: the development of large central computers, the appearance of microcomputers that replaced passive terminals, the development of mini-computers tied together into distributed systems, and more recently the development of wide-area networks and Internet-based applications. HIS boundaries have been extended to multisite environments and more recently to the community under the broader concept of community health information systems (CHISs) or networks (CHINs).

Although several dozen products are on the market, few of them actually cover all the requirements of healthcare institutions and provide the adequate integration into the larger healthcare networks. The diversity of the tasks to be performed, the players involved, the existing organizations, and the technical possibilities explain this situation.

This book focuses on clinical information systems (CISs), considered as the subsystem of CHISs that are devoted to the direct management of the patient. It represents to CHISs what clinical informatics is to medical or health informatics. The subtitle *A Component-Based Approach* stresses the idea that an integrated and comprehensive CIS can be built up from a basic set of interdependent components. This approach, which finds its background in modern software engineering, should help in building up more flexible and adaptable systems in a domain where technology is changing very rapidly.

This book is designed for all healthcare professionals involved in the design, development, evolution, or distribution of open CISs. Decision makers have to face important alternatives that need to consider functionalities, evolutivity, and costs. HIS architects will concentrate on the optimal definition of and collaboration between components. The book does not require any specialized mathematical or statistical knowledge.

The first chapter shows the evolution of CISs from a functional, a technical, and an architectural perspective. Chapters 2 and 3 consider CISs as a collection of collaborative business objects. An architecture around six basic components is presented. Chapters 4 to 9 describe each basic component in detail. Chapter 10 describes the specific aspects of the integration of PACS and CIS. In Chapters 11 to 14, four case studies relate experiences in the development and/or deployment of component-based CISs: the AZ-VUB in Brussels, the Pompidou University Hospital in Paris, the Cantonal University Hospital in Geneva, and the Vanderbilt University Hospital in Nashville. The principal technical terms used in clinical informatics and software engineering and their definitions may be found in the glossary.

A number of people have provided comments and criticism, and we would particularly like to thank Françoise Aimé, Elisabeth Delbecke, Marion Lavril-Robey, and Lise Marin. When we were preparing this textbook, Marion J. Ball and Kathryn J. Hannah nicely encouraged us. We are indebted to them for their warm and constant support. Anne Tomasino greatly helped us with the Shakespearean language.

Rudi Van de Velde
Patrice Degoulet

Contents

10 Imaging Management and Integration 191

11 AZ-VUB Clinical Information System 217

Rudi Van de Velde, Rony Lanssiers, Goedele Antonissen,
and Vital Claeys

1

Introduction: The Evolution of Health Information Systems

The real voyage of discovery consists not in seeking new landscapes, but in having new eyes.
—Marcel Proust

Today healthcare professionals expect to access lifelong patient records that are created by linking multiple encounters, adapting knowledge and decision tools to support prevention, prediction, and care. This is the result of the long history of development of medical information systems whose origin can be found in the early 1960s. This chapter summarizes the evolution of information systems from both a functional and a technical perspective.

Functional Perspective

Hospital Information Systems

Since their early beginning in the 1960s, *hospital information systems* (HISs) have been developed to cover both administrative and medical functions [Collen 1999]. However, it must be recognized that the first systems often focused on the billing and reimbursement aspects of hospital activities. These systems were designed to provide a money-oriented return on investment (get the money) and streamline patient admissions. They managed appointments and provided (stand-alone) ancillary services for hospital laboratories, the pharmacy, and radiology departments. They were developed to support existing manual procedures without adding value, and they functioned as a bonding element among the many disparate systems inside and outside the hospital. They improved accuracy and were supposed to save time for personnel.

The 1980s saw the implementation of two nearly worldwide changes with a significant impact on the way computer applications were used in hospitals.

On one hand, reimbursement systems gradually evolved from a fee-for-service basis to a fixed budget system where figures on resource consumption played a central role. On the other hand, medical systems initially developed to simply automate existing processes became systems supporting physicians, nurses, and other healthcare providers in their daily patient care activities. The aim was to attempt to guarantee standards of care and lead to improved levels of decision making (Figure 1.1).

In early HISs, resource consumption and allocation were only roughly measured by length of stay. The usefulness of data originating from these systems was limited. Because of the significant variance between hospitals, it was impossible to compare one hospital's data with another's. Today, as patients and payers demand evidence of quality of care and cost reduction, it is obvious that these types of indicators are insufficient, and hospitals seek other competitive metrics such as process outcome measurements. The answers to many questions could be found only in reams of mostly hand-written paper-based clinical notes. The need for clinical information systems became obvious. It is more and more necessary for physicians to achieve targeted standards of care, from a quality and cost perspective, and for hospital administrators to gain some level of control over the behavior of clinicians [Clayton 1997].

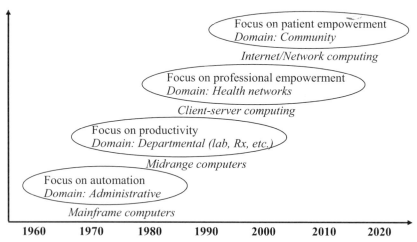

Figure 1.1: Changing destiny of information technology in the health sector.

Community Health Information Systems

Cooperative and/or *community health information systems* (CHISs) or *networks* (CHINs) arise as technologies accelerate and opportunities to exchange and share data become wider, and because patients living in the "global village" become more and more mobile (Figure 1.2).

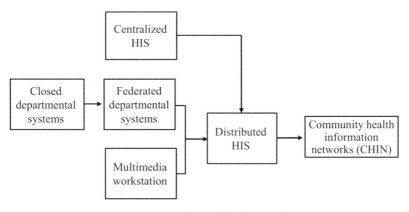

Figure 1.2: Evolution of hospital information systems.

A CHIS (or CHIN) provides comprehensive and integrated sets of health care and information services between primary and secondary care institutions, social and administrative institutions, and it offers on-line information resources for education and training. Community-wide data networking and sharing in health care is characterized by a huge flow between various institutions of three main types of information: patient data (patient characteristics, health status, risk behavior, resource use), administrative data (medical care outcomes), and scientific and educational data. Each has different standards, security requirements, and integration needs. Despite the progress in information technology, information exchanges are still performed in most countries via classical mail, courier, and fax, and local applications are rarely integrated in communication systems. CHISs may have a tremendous impact on health care, provide a more detailed picture of patient health, and enhance the analysis of the health of the communities served by these systems [Showstack 1996]. The creation of effective community health information networks depends on willingness to share data.

Clinical Information Systems

In the 1990s, it became clear that the objective of reducing expenditures could be achieved only by creating information systems that assist physicians in their daily care activities (decision-making features) and also integrate resource consumption and allocation. The development of clinical information systems (CISs) was a natural evolution within the HIS and CHIS frameworks in order to expand their functions to include better management of patient care.

The issue of whether information is administrative or clinical is no longer relevant in the era of an integrated healthcare enterprise where users require access to all types of information and services. CISs are driven by an economic and medical motivation to achieve quality of care combined with an increased level of control. As these functions cannot originate from a single vendor, every institution or group of institutions must define the information architecture that integrates this heterogeneity. Moreover, as no one vendor can cover the broad scope of the various applications necessary, integration expertise (delivered in house or available outside) is very important.

Technology Perspective

The two most promising developments that may have a mass impact on the development of healthcare information systems are the emergence of component-driven technologies on one hand, and the importance of mobile communications on the other [Kleinberg 1998].

Object-Oriented and Component-Based Computing

The worlds of *distributed computing* and *object-oriented computing* have evolved separately but are actually symbiotic in nature. Each world shares several core concepts, as indicated in Figure 1.3. The words are different, but the meanings are essentially the same, the intersection of both worlds leading to the world of componentry.

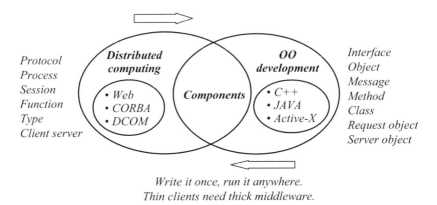

Write it once, run it anywhere.
Thin clients need thick middleware.

Figure 1.3: Componentry: The intersection of two dynamic forces.

Component-based technologies foster the evolution from a data-driven to a knowledge-driven architecture. They allow embedding the organization's knowledge practices and policies into business rules located in the component layer. They facilitate the maintenance and scalability of complex applications, thus increasing their long-term viability (Figure 1.4). A component is a software unit living on a node. It is a physical implementation of a set of logical elements (such as classes and collaborations), that provides the realization of a set of interfaces [Herzum 2000].

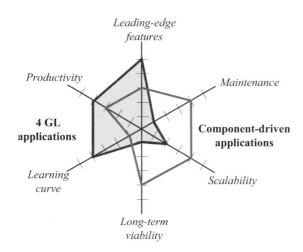

Figure 1.4: A comparison of the development approaches. The scale ranges from
1 = bad to 5 = excellent. 4 GL: fourth-generation language.

Middleware

In a world of component-based applications, middleware will take an important place (Figure 1.5). The concept of middleware is rather fuzzy. The term "middleware" can be applied at its simplest to EDI (electronic data interchange) and asynchronous modes of communication. Client/server middleware systems provide synchronous communication between senders and receivers. MOM message oriented middleware) is a class of middleware that provides message passing and queuing between systems but is implemented on an asynchronous basis [Myerson 2002].

According to Spahni et al. [Spahni 1998], three categories of middleware can be established in the healthcare domain on the basis of the services they provide:

- *First-generation elementary middleware* originated in the mid-1980s. It enhances the portability of applications over different platforms. It refers to remote procedure calls (RPC) and enables applications to call other systems. This generation of middleware deserves to be mentioned, although various widely accepted incompatible RPC implementations exist (e.g., Sun RPC, distributed computing environment RPC, OSI RPC, and so on).

- *Second-generation middleware* is characterized by an increased availability of other services (resource localization over the network, resource management, and so on) and refers to ORBs (object request brokers). They allow distributed objects to be managed in a very flexible way. Examples are CORBA (Common Object Request Broker) and Microsoft COM/DCOM.

Third-generation middleware provides generic services to applications tailored within a specific application domain. These systems are at the more sophisticated end of the middleware range. The goal is to offer a broad number of services that enable users to build and tailor their own applications. Examples are CORBAmed and the CEN TC251 HISA (healthcare information system architecture) that introduced two groups of services: generic common services (GCS) and health specific common services (HCS). Another example based on the HISA specification is provided by the HANSA consortium as DHE (distributed healthcare environment) [Ferrara 1998].

Emerging technology	Description	Underlying technology	Challenges
Component-based technologies			
Object-based middleware	• Software that allows objects or components to cooperate	• Application servers (J2EE, DCOM) • Object-request brokers (ORBs) • Transaction-processing monitors	• Cultural change • Scalability • Lack of development and management tools
Mobile communications			
Portable computers	• Notebooks • Hand-held • Tablet PC • PDAs • PDA phone	• Special-device operating systems (Windows CE, Palm OS, ...) • Special-purpose hardware	• Weight • Battery lifetime • Wireless communication features
Wireless data communications	• Analog (radio-based) or digital • Local or wide-area network communication	• Wireless LAN (IEEE 802.11), Bluetooth • WAP, GPRS, UMTS • Wireless Internet	• Bandwidth • Geographic coverage • Interference
Intelligent software layers			
Intelligent software	• Intelligent software layer that can react to the environment	• Rule-based techniques • Software agents	• Performance • Standards (maintenance) • Software reuse

Figure 1.5: Emerging technology challenges. WAP: Wireless Access Protocol; UMTS: Universal Mobile Telecommunications System; GPRS: General Packet Radio Service; PDA: Personal Digital Assistant.

Mobile Communications

Personal digital assistants and wireless technologies bring computing to disconnected workers, a group that seldom has the inclination to type or the ability to lug around unwieldy devices (Figure 1.5). They require advances in user interfaces, reliability, power consumption, and miniaturization. Last but not least, wireless communication technologies will foster access to data at any point of care both locally and remotely. Intelligent messaging based on workflow (group) technologies and fast information bus structures support the strong communication character of health care.

Architectural Perspective

Mainframe Architectures

Although all information systems were affected by the remarkable expansion in computer technology, it is clear that the progress implemented by health institutions was not as significant as that implemented by other industries.

From the 1960s to the early 1980s, the computer industry was basically vertically aligned. This meant that a respectable computer company developed its own chips, own computers, own/proprietary OS and very often proprietary application software. The physical platform was centralized in one location. All the data were consolidated in one database. All subject databases were interrelated and physically stored on the same server. This helped to maximize the available processing power.

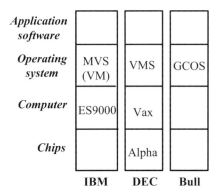

Figure 1.6: Vertically oriented computer industry in the 1980s.

Mainframe systems, ideal in an era of centralized organizations, led to successful transaction processing systems capable of supporting many online users, but they were difficult to use and expensive to modify and maintain.

This vertically aligned industry offered maximum integration at the expense of the tight coupling, over a long period, of users to one computer company. It was not possible to discard just one part of the vertical stack; the user had to abandon the entire stack (Figure 1.6). In addition, these monolithic systems were mainly administration driven and characterized by cumbersome and proprietary user interfaces.

Departmental Systems

The second wave of information systems centered on the development of departmental systems, many of which are still in use in hospitals today. This departmental approach is commonly defined in the literature as a federated architecture. Information was frequently distributed by application domains, for example, financial data on a server at one site, patient data at another node, laboratory data at another node, and so on. Medically oriented applications appeared, notably in the field of clinical laboratories, pharmacy, radiology, and order entry and communication. From the point of view of software development, everything that was built was monolithic.

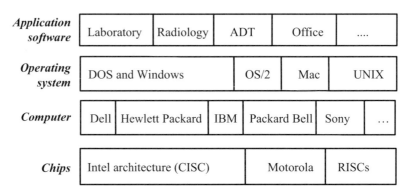

Figure 1.7: Horizontally oriented computer industry in the 1990s.

In the 1980s with the appearance of microprocessor chips, manufacturing computers became extremely cost-effective (high volume, low cost) and gave birth to the minicomputer and personal computer. In the meantime the entire computer industry gradually shifted away from vertical alignment. A new "horizontal" computer industry emerged (Figure 1.7).

The strengths of the vertical wave became the weaknesses of the horizontal computer industry; dealing with various vendors and various products (components) that require seamless interworking.

Distributed Systems and the Client/Server Era

In a distributed environment, applications are basically composed of interoperable components: data objects, application objects (managing the business processes), and user interfaces. Applications objects were removed from the mainframe to build up client/server (C/S) architectures (Figure 1.8). At least three driving forces led to the concept of client/server architectures:

- ease of use and consistency sought by users when they use GUIs,
- high degree of autonomy in manipulating data, and
- belief that PCs attached to inexpensive servers offer better price/performance at reduced cost.

For the most part, this was true even if difficulties that did not previously exist on the mainframe were observed: increased client management on a large number of PCs and increased network traffic that is difficult to scale.

Many distribution schemes ranging from thick-client to thin-client systems are described in the literature [Stonebraker 1998]. Currently the most popular system is the monolithic thick-client system, where all code is located on the client side, resulting in the so-called thick-client distribution scheme. A thick-client application needs to make multiple calls to a database in order to populate itself so that it can manipulate the data (Figure 1.8).

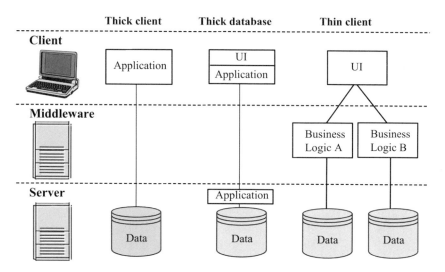

Figure 1.8: Three places business logic can reside.

In thick-database architecture, a thin-client makes a single call to a thick database. The thick database acts as its own application server, performing data manipulations while the data is still in the database. It then returns the data to the client.

To regain the benefits of centralized architectures, the business logic can be transferred from the client to an intermediate layer, giving birth to "three-tier" architecture. In this architecture, a thin client makes a call to an application server, possibly located close to the database, even on the same machine, or makes multiple calls to the database to get the information the client wants. It off loads processing from central servers, retains many of the advantages of a centralized mainframe, has reduced client management requirements, and scales well. The disadvantages are performance penalties since traffic increases with an increased number of communicating nodes (systems).

In the event of a large installed base of workstations in a thin-client distribution scheme, a message broker system might be the preferred choice. It would ease the management of the peripherals, but it would increase network traffic.

Network-Centric Architectures and Web Services

With the explosive development of the Internet, application components can be made ubiquitously available. Web services provide this functionality. A Web service is a network-accessible piece of business logic, located somewhere on the Internet, and accessible through standard based Internet technologies (HTTP, XML, SMTP) [Cauld 2002, Snell 2002]. Web services are able to act as a mediator tool for sending and receiving messages [Chappell 2002]. The data carried around the network by the transport layer can be packaged in an HTML format strongly related to the presentation logic or in the SOAP extension of the XML specification. Web services are platform-independent, firewall-friendly, and inherently loosely coupled.

Several technologies are emerging as worldwide standards that make up the code of today's Web services technology:

- SOAP, the Simple Object Access Protocol, specifies a standard packaging structure for transporting XML documents over a variety of standard Internet technologies, including SMTP, HTTP, and FTP. A SOAP message consists of an envelope for the information being transferred within the message, and contains an (optional) header and a required body. SOAP defines a set of encoding rules for translating application and platform-specific data types into XML representations.

- WSDL, the Web Service Description Language, is an XML-based language that describes the interface of a Web service in a standardized way. It provides a contract between a Web service and the outside world.

- UDDI, the Universal Description, Discovery, and Integration initiative, provides a worldwide registry of Web services for publishing, discovery, and integration purposes.

- BPML, the Business Process Modeling Language, is a metalanguage for the modeling of business processes.

The relationship between SOAP, WSDL, and UDDI is summarized in Figure 1.9. An application (a Web service client) needs to locate another application or a piece of business logic located somewhere on the network. The client queries a UDDI registry (server) for the service either by name, category, identifier, or specification supported. Once located, the client obtains information about the location of a WSDL document from the UDDI registry. The WSDL document outlines what messages this SOAP server expects in

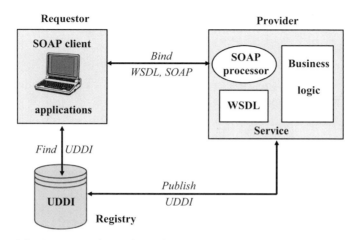

Figure 1.9: Anatomy of a Web service. A Web service consists of several key components. SOAP: Simple Object Access Protocol; UDDI: Universal Universal Description, Discovery, and Integration initiative; WSDL: Web Service Description Language.

order to provide services, as well as what messages it returns. The client creates a SOAP message in accordance with the XML schema found in the WSDL and sends a request to the host (where the service is).

Toward Component-Based Clinical Information Systems

For years the debate has focused on the optimum architecture of clinical information systems. The target architecture should be modular and driven by the size of the implementation and the institution requirements for scalability, availability, and systems management.

Component-based and *N*-tier architectures may become the enterprise computing standard for the coming years. A component-based approach enables scalable, cost-effective three- or *N*-tier hardware deployment. Scaling can occur in either the middle layer or the data layer in a much less expensive manner. It provides

- ways of achieving enhanced load balancing;
- flexibility of application partitioning for power, performance, and/or management;
- enabled embedment of decision support for business logic;
- complete upgrade, from a maintenance point of view, of the business logic software performed at one or more server locations and instantaneously affecting hundreds of viewing stations (changes are isolated to fewer tiers);

- easier integration of heterogeneous resources;
- service longevity (it is more flexible and adaptable in meeting changing business needs than traditional client/server technologies); and
- easier reuse of components, as well as code.

However, component-based and *N*-tier systems can be annoyingly complex for the following reasons:

- An *N*-tier architecture causes a complex design and development phase. Therefore, it requires education, discipline, and skills from programmers.
- There are too many choices, most with consequences (the good of the many versus the good of the one).
- Complex management and deployment are likely.
- Tool insertion is associated with increasing costs. When a problem occurs in a distributed environment, any of the intervening pieces may be incriminated.
- Incompatibilities between diverse software and hardware components originating from multiple vendors may occur.
- Performance pitfalls can be the case as additional layers or components are added, hence additional performance monitoring is needed.

The phrase "Keep it simple, stupid" remains true. Therefore component-based computing has to be an exercise in minimalism, limiting the number of components, protocols, and standards that are deployed [Carner 1994]. Learning to cope with complexity and to handle all the problems is also a part of the training required.

Summary and Conclusions

If we were to assign names to the recent decades in general computing terms, the 1970s would be the decade of monolithic applications centered around proprietary mainframes, the 1980s the decade of federated systems composed of loosely coupled systems, and the 1990s would be the decade of distributed applications [Stonebraker 1998]. Concurrently, there was an emphasis on data and knowledge integration in earlier days giving rise to data warehouses and decision support systems.

The first wave of information processing in health care dealt with automating administrative processes. The second focused on medical departmental applications, but it covered only a limited number of application domains since the systems had to be created at the source with the aim of literally replacing manual systems.

Administrative and basic medical functions in hospitals today are highly computerized, and a significant number of vertical commercial systems are available on the market. They are characterized by rich functionalities that may often conflict with each other or are redundant with data acquisition applications, for example. Their main drawbacks are the fact that they are difficult and expensive to adapt to new requirements and to integrate with existing systems.

We are now entering the era of real medically oriented information systems that encourage integration of all existing satellite systems (external and internal) into one coherent, interoperable environment around electronic health records (EHR). This wave of information processing divides the system into parts based on a specific property: data activity, function, geographical location, and so on.

The most effective way of preventing medical errors is to prevent them at the point and time of care. This is possible using modern information technology such as mobile terminals, electronic health records, alerts-and-reminders systems, which alert health professionals when, for example, the patient is allergic to the medication that has just been ordered. Such computer systems can also greatly improve efficiency and reduce costs. Technology and business life cycles are becoming shorter. They impose new requirements, provide new opportunities, and give rise to new expectations. The implementation of each new technology will affect health care organizations and administrative regulations as shown in Figure 1.10. Health professional users try, in fact, to get the most from their information systems. We must beware of becoming overenthusiastic at the announcement of new technologies that are still in infancy. It should be stressed that technology is not a panacea but a tool, often an expensive one, designed to enhance human interaction. In the clinical field, the appropriate technology must match the applications.

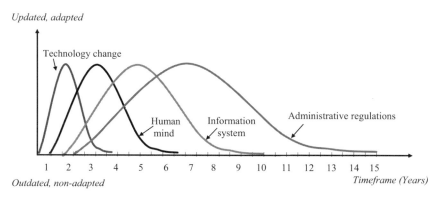

Figure 1.10: Impact of technology change on human mind, organizations, and administrative regulations.

Optimal management of the requirements for health care urge us to take another look at the user/clinical information system relationship. Although we have witnessed a remarkable growth in computer technology in hospitals, most existing systems remain vertically organized and characterized by the duplication of data and functionalities dispersed over various applications, which prevents data sharing. Component technology requires greater collaboration and coordination.

References

[Carner 1994] Carner R. Unsupportable costs. *Open Computing.* 1994; 11(2): 35–41.

[Cauld 2002] Cauldwell P, Chawla R, Chopra V, Damschen G, Dix C, Hong T, Norton F, Ogbuji U, Olander G, Richman M, Saunders K, Zaev Z. *Professional XML Web services.* Birmingham: Wrox Press, 2002.

[Chappell 2002] Chappell DA, Jewell T. *Java Web Services.* Sebastopol: O'Reilly; 2002.

[Clayton 1997] Clayton PD, Van Mulligen EM. Hospital information systems: Clinical. In: *Handbook of Medical Informatics.* Van Bemmel JH, Musen MA (editors). Heidelberg: Springer-Verlag. 1997; 331–341.

[Collen 1970] Collen MF. General requirements for a medical information system (MIS). *Comput Biomed Res.* 1970; 3(5): 393–406.

[Collen 1991] Collen MF. A brief historical overview of hospital information system (HIS) evolution in the United States. *Int J Biomed Comput.* 1991; 29(3–4): 169–189.

[Collen 1999] Collen MF. The evolution of computer communications. *MD Comput.* 1999;16 (4): 72–76.

[Ferrara 1998] Ferrara FM. The standard healthcare information systems architecture and the DHE middleware. *Int J Med Inform.* 1998; 52(1–3): 39–51.

[Hripcsak 1997] Hripcsak G. IAIMS architecture. *J Am Med Inform Assoc.* 1997; 4 (2 Suppl): S20–S30.

[Kleinberg 1998] Kleinberg K. *Advanced Architectures in Healthcare: Technology Hurdles.* Technical report T-03-4484. Gartner Group. Jan 13 1998.

[Myers 2002] Myers JM. *The Complete Book of Middleware.* Boca Raton, FL: Auerbach, 2002.

[Showstack 1996] Showstack J, Lurie N, Leatherman S, Fisher E, Inui T. Health of the Public: The private-sector challenge. *JAMA.* 1996; 276 (13): 1071–1074.

[Snell 2002] Snell J, Tidwell D, Kulchenko P. *Programming Web Services with SOAP.* Sebastopol, CA: O'Reilly, 2002.

[Spahni 1998] Spahni S, Scherrer JR, Sauquet D, Sottile PA. Middleware for healthcare information systems. *Medinfo.* 1998; 9 Pt 1: 212–216.

[Stonebraker 1998] Stonebraker M. Betting on ORDBMS. *Byte.* 1998; 23 (4): 91–96.

2

Frameworks: A Collection of Business Objects

A New Vision

Off-the-shelf computer systems are not always an ideal alternative to in-house built-in systems. It is indeed difficult to find a package that fits all the needs of a health institution. Moreover, the hidden costs involved in customizing a package to integrate it into an existing environment is often outrageous or unknown. There seems to be a trend toward customizing less rather than too much. Major vendors are providing "model" systems to which many early adopters and heavy customers are reverting, often causing unintended effects and maintenance difficulties. On the other hand, custom-made products are disappearing and are gradually being replaced by the assembly of prebuilt reusable components. As software development is similar to the production process of highly sophisticated industrial products, the ultimate goal should be to deliver maintainable and reusable building blocks. Architectures based on components reduce development costs, allow the replacement of components, and finally enable differentiation through customizing. Whenever possible, developers must (re)use existing software components to solve problems that are not related to their domain. In the medical field they should try to reduce the complexity of the medical applications development process and concentrate on the business aspects that ultimately represent the added value of their applications [IBM 1998].

The increasing complexity of medical applications and the need to maintain a high degree of extensibility and at the same time the need to deliver reliable and robust software can be addressed by applying a number of key concepts such as abstraction, decomposition, layering, and iteration. The technique of decomposition, dividing a complex problem into smaller, manageable units, each of which can then be accomplished separately, is the core of component-based development (CBD) [Herzum 2000]. This evolution of application development has also been driven by advances in computer technology and the penetration of Internet and intranet technologies that has changed the way users think about access to information.

Components cover a wide range varying from technological to general and domain-specific aspects [Cummins 2002]. If we analyze commercial admission-discharge-transfer (ADT) systems today, a very large number of functions are the same. The local organization of healthcare services differentiates these packages. Hence, software developers must concentrate on understanding the specific (industry) subdomains together with the corresponding local and cultural requirements.

Before going into more detail, it is important to emphasize that the implementation of any information system follows a logical process from concept definition through requirements and design before arriving at implementation (Figure 2.1).

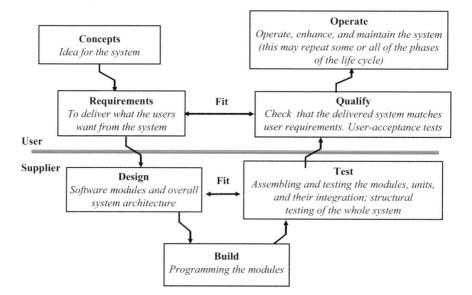

Figure 2.1: The software development life cycle.

Software Components

There is much discussion about components versus objects and the relationship that exists between them. Software objects are a way to represent the universe of discourse. A software object can be a tangible thing, an idea, or an event. Objects are unique, so they are defined by an identifier. They provide a number of services and allow the manipulation of data in the object. They are made visible to the outside world by means of an interface. The implementation or a description of how the object works is hidden. The implementation consists of data and code (Figure 2.2). Many objects can share the same implementation [Brown 2000]. An object can have many interfaces or many objects can share the same interface.

Components are predefined building blocks, packaging one or more objects (implementations) designed so that developers can construct systems even with no knowledge of the component's implementation details. Components come in two different "flavors," horizontal and vertical. *Horizontal components* can be reused enterprise-wide across multiple projects and multiple application domains. Examples of horizontal components include generalized collection classes, persistent storage classes, application framework classes, and design patterns. *Vertical components* are domain-specific, and therefore are typically encoded with a great deal of knowledge that is local to the application services being developed. Commercial class libraries are widely available for both types of components.

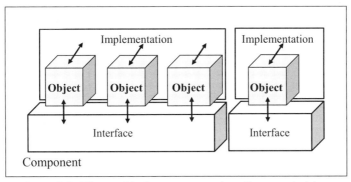

Figure 2.2: The world of components, interfaces, and objects.

A component is based on a *component model* or *framework*. A component model provides a number of services that support the software and a number of rules to be obeyed by the component complying with that model to take advantage of the services. Well-known component models include Sun's JavaBeans and Enterprise JavaBeans (EJB), the OMG's emerging CORBA component standard, and Microsoft's COM+. Each of these component models determines how a component makes its services available to others, how components are named, and how new components and their services are discovered at runtime. The continuing growth of component software in the years ahead must answer increasing user demand with a limited pool of available software skills.

Component software development consists of building applications from reusable parts and plugging them into some kind of container or framework instead of building large applications (Figure 2.3). It reflects the emerging network-centric computing models; it is a more flexible way to create customized software solutions and revise and use software so that it works the way people do. It is assumed that the best way to build large-scale systems is to break down systems into their functional components [Herzum 2000].

Frameworks define the architecture of an application and regulate the collaboration between the collection of its business objects. More precisely, frameworks

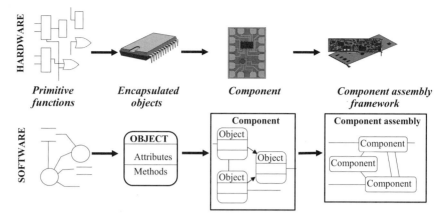

Figure 2.3: Components and frameworks in the world of hardware and software.

- define rules that objects need to follow to resemble their real-world counterpart objects,
- allow data exchange and handle all the control flow,
- allow the exchange of services between objects by messaging,
- provide a consistent execution environment, and
- are a container for business objects.

A framework takes care of all flow control and calls the programmer's code only when necessary [Bohrer 1998]. The key difference between *frameworks* and *components* is that frameworks are sold to developers, while components are ready to use and provided to end users.

There are at least three interrelated reasons why a component architecture might become the enterprise computing standard:

- Component software architectures are more flexible and adaptable in meeting changing business needs than traditional client/server architectures.
- Component software enables scalable three- or N-tier hardware deployment. Scaling can now occur, through a set of tricks such as database multiplexing and load balancing [Linthicum 1999], in either the middle layer or the data layer in a much less expensive manner.
- Component systems have lower total cost of ownership in complex enterprises. By placing some or most of the application logic on a middle tier, the developer has better control over the application logic.

Software Objects

According to the OMG's business object management special interest group (BOMSIG), a *business object* (defining the model) is a representation of a thing active in the business domain, including at least its business name and definition, attributes, behavior, relationship, and constraints. A business object represents, for example, a patient, an order, a ward unit, or a concept [OMG 1997]. Business objects describe application-independent concepts and encapsulate storage, metadata, and *business rules* associated with the real perceivable entities [Orfali 1997, 1999]. Business objects do not exist in isolation. They need to collaborate with other business objects.

A second type of object is *presentation objects* (defining the view) that represent a visual metaphor on the screen to end users and provide them with the features necessary to work and communicate with the business model.

A third type of object is *business process* (defining the control) or *application objects*. They are nonpersistent, control the logic of the process, and encapsulate business logic. In fact this is a variation of the controller part in the *model/view/controller* (MVC) paradigm of Smalltalk that defines the way the user interface reacts to the user input and *graphical user interface* (GUI) events [Bohrer 1998, Orfali 1999]. The model corresponds with the business object layer that persists at a business server and interacts with services that provide persistence (database server). The view, a proxy of the model, is visible and accessible to a user on a client workstation. The controller embodies transaction services and specifies all collaboration patterns between business objects. It accepts triggers from the view and breaks them down into messages for the server below.

Objects relate to each other in three different ways:
- by specialization or generalization,
- by composition, and
- by collaboration.

Business Rules

Business rules are the natural language expressions every organization uses to state its practices and policies. By concentrating on the business rules and processes in a middle tier, three-tier architectures represent a natural solution to these problems. Traditional information systems become obsolete as requirements hence business rules—traditionally buried deep in procedural code—change. This approach makes these systems inflexible and inconsistent, and makes rapid changes virtually impossible.

Business rules can be grouped into two major classes: structure-based and declarative rules [Usoft 1998]. Structure-based rules are inherent in and defined through the business (object) model itself. Examples of structure-based rules follow:
- Patients must have at least one order.
- A date is mandatory for each transaction and cannot be changed.
- A patient cannot be deleted if he has outstanding results.

Declarative rules contain more complex business logic than can be defined through the object model. Their behavior exists in conjunction with structure-based rules. Declarative rules can be further broken down into restrictive and corrective rules. Restrictive rules prevent conditions from ever becoming true in the business. Corrective rules make changes to the data based on conditions occurring.

Constraints are examples of declarative rules. They include

- restrictive constraints (e.g., patients are not allowed to have more than one computed tomography within 24 hours) and

- corrective constraints (e.g., if a patient has taken all the medication from one specific medication order, a reorder is generated automatically).

Architectural Requirements

The development of a healthcare information infrastructure is an exercise in managing complexity. A lot of architectural work has been done in this area (e.g., in the Cosmos, RICHE, and Edith projects [IMG 1992, RICHE 1992, Ferrara 1998], or by the CEN PT013 group), but little work was based on a component-driven philosophy. Driven by the increased complexity of health-care organizations and by the different technology rates observed on various subsystems, an architectural framework must respond to the following requirements [Tskiknakis 1997]:

Interoperability between multiple specialized, distributed or existing legacy systems. The design should support particular data types and business functions located in separate information systems. It should improve the coordination, shareability, and reusability of information between various departments within a large clinical environment where patients are nowadays frequently treated independently for different problems [Hammond 1994]. Interoperability requires not only information sharing but also collaboration through connectivity between healthcare actors and systems. To be able to schedule, initiate, monitor, and control predefined administrative and clinical procedures, a workflow management system providing the ability to cooperate in performing tasks is necessary [Leisch 1997].

Heterogeneity of information sources and platforms. A healthcare organization has multiple distributed repositories with patient-related information spread over departmental systems. Each departmental system is responsible for the creation and tracking of its own data. Integrating these diverse medical applications, written in different languages on incompatible systems over a range of networks, is a challenging problem. This integration does not simply involve connecting systems or departments. Its aim is also to achieve an organizational integration. The architecture must provide an interface on the technical and logical levels with all departmental systems to identify which information must be exchanged and the way it should happen. On the logical level, a common understanding is necessary to overcome differences in notations used (in terms of registered data, vocabularies, codifications, and so on).

User-interface consistency and homogeneity. On the presentation level, a consistent and homogeneous user interface that is compliant with the user needs and privileges strongly reduces the learning curve. Furthermore, differentiation through customizing for variations in customer business processes must be available.

Scalability and extensibility are needed to maintain local ownership of data in order to cover new aspects of the healthcare domain as the system grows.

Accessibility and adaptability. On the functional level, users and clinicians, depending on their profile, must have access to core medical functions such as clinical decision support systems, the latest medical literature, order entry, patient demographics, e-mail, results reporting, alerts, reminders, and so on.

Architectural Design

Architecture Layers

The information requirements of an organization can be examined from two distinct but interrelated angles: the logical and the physical architecture of a system. The logical architecture emphasizes the business model synchronized with the institutional requirements, the application model defining the environment in which business objects are used, and the way users interface with the system. The physical architecture of the system deals with the technical infrastructure: the distribution scheme of software and hardware among the nodes, file systems elected, and networks.

The logical architecture is organized vertically into horizontal layers and horizontally into vertical subsystems referred to in the literature as functional areas, frameworks, or components. Functional areas are "vertical" in the sense that all the classes that represent a rather independent group of coherent, autonomous decision-making and function-oriented entities belong to one subsystem [IBM 1998, Wilson 1999]. A healthcare organization carries out specific functions related to healthcare delivery. Hence a healthcare information system based on user profiles may be clustered in homogeneous groups of activities and data that correspond with component.

There is an important difference between class libraries and business components (Figure 2.4). An *application* uses a set of components to provide and support the requirements and activities of a specific functional area or an individual unit in the organization. *Service functions* are provided by one component to other components of the health information system. Each service can be invoked by any component of the system through a formal mech-

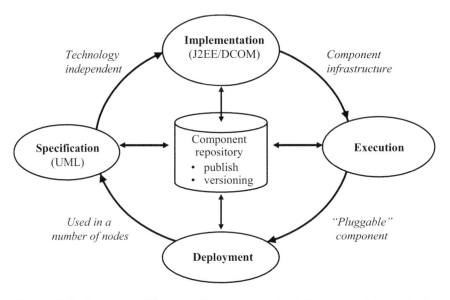

Figure 2.4: Component life cycle. The process of building, managing, and using
software components. UML: Unified Modeling Language.

anism and documented according to a formal and unambiguous syntax,
depending on the programming languages supported.

By partitioning the system into layers it is easier to cope with a constantly
evolving health environment and modify one layer without making modifications to the other layers. Layers can be designed using a bottom-up approach
(from business to view). However, to achieve the highest degree of freedom
and expressiveness, the development of a particular layer should not be hin-
dered by the layer that is above.

Three distinct layers can be considered: a *view (application) layer* as part
of the application domain, a *persistent storage* layer, and a *business layer*.The
persistent layer corresponds to the file system in use. It is responsible for
storing the objects in some form of persistent storage.The business layer identifies two different kinds of objects:

- Objects that model recognizable everyday life entities and correspond to
  named classes. They are often referred to in the literature as *business
  objects* and behave like nouns in sentences.

- *Business process objects* (sometimes defined as application objects in
  the literature) that make up the foundation of the application and view
  layer above. They also explain how an object reacts to changes in the
  views or in the model and are independent of any application. They
  behave like verbs in sentences.

There are three basic goals for the existence of the business layer [Monday
1998]:

- Objects are used across multiple vertical domains (subsystems).

- Interfaces allow vertical domains to communicate with each other and with legacy applications.
- Objects and design patterns are useful to the vertical domains.

There is no standard health institution or hospital service model. It is therefore preferable to define a collection of standard components that various medical applications might use and on which healthcare players might agree. These collections of business objects, endorsed within a structure, encapsulate persistent business data–metadata and their behavior (individual process definitions) evolves over time. They convey knowledge and support the fundamental requirements of the domain in particular and the healthcare organization in general in terms of

- information processed,
- activities performed and services delivered, and
- communication and cooperation capabilities.

Business objects do not specifically belong to a particular application but focus on the core clinical business processes. Every business component relates to a particular business domain. It is very generic and identifiable by users and programmers of the organization and might be used by various applications. For example, components identified as core business components in a medical environment are patients, activities, and health data.

Components are characterized as highly reusable and are mostly persistent. They may correspond to healthcare-related or generic services, as defined by the project team PT013 (WG1) of the CEN, the European standardization committee, in a document entitled a *Standard Architecture for Health care Information Systems* [CEN 1997b]. This model has been extended and modified [Van de Velde 1997]. Within the business layer of this model, two types of components can be identified. The *healthcare common components* (HCC) support the processes and information relevant to the health care domain. The *generic* (business) *common components* (GCC) support the functions common to any type of business domain.

The view layer, sometimes referred to as the application layer, implements the application logic and its behavior and maintains status information on the current use of the system (e.g., the currently selected patient, the selected results). The application domain represents the highest degree of specialization vertically supporting the specific needs of individual healthcare units (nodes) that represent coherent and autonomous decision-making entities. The application layer requests services from the underlying business layer. It may contain business process classes that mediate between the view layer and the business layer. The application layer provides the environment to execute the business objects. This layer is process-oriented, encapsulates the business logic and acts as the glue between the other objects.

For example, the business layer models the relationship between a patient and his or her medical history as a one-to-many relationship, while the view layer, when requested by a cardiologist, will only show the cardiovascular history of the patient ignoring the other historical data. The application designer considers the different healthcare business components implemented by the framework and highlights the components that need to be customized according to the application domain requirements. Programmers implement the requirements by extending, modifying, or aggregating existing classes in the application layer.

Dynamics of the Architecture

Three independent models can be used to represent the architecture of any specific technological environment. The *static model* of the components provides descriptions (in terms of attributes and attribute values) and shows relationships between components (associations, aggregations, or generalizations). The *dynamic model* provides graphical notations for events, event traces, states, state transitions, and hierarchies of states. It explains how various classes act together in specific scenarios. The *functional model* completes the composite model. Since objects (data) were defined in the object model and behavior was defined in the dynamic model, the only thing left to be defined in the functional model are actions (operations, processes, or functions) and constraints on actions.

Object interactions can be captured and described using popular design methodology tools such as the UML notation [Booch 1999] that unifies former methodologies such as Rumbaugh's *event traces* [Rumbaugh 1991], Graham's *task scripts* [Graham 1995], Booch's *interaction diagrams* [Booch 1994], and Jacobson's *use cases* [Jacobson 1992].

Enterprise Infostructure Model

This section provides the strategic specification (the logical or enterprise-level model) of the healthcare-related business components of the healthcare information system. Healthcare business components support the fundamental requirements of healthcare organizations in terms of information processed, activities performed, and services delivered together with the provision of communication and cooperation facilities. The set of business components is nevertheless to be considered open, in the sense that it can be extended with additional architectural elements. The architecture evolves over time by taking into account the evolution of requirements significant for the whole organization.

From a strategic point of view, the essence of any healthcare environment can be described by the following sentence:

> A medical organization consists of *authorized agents* who perform *activities* related to the need of a *subject of care* using *resources* and generating an *outcome* based on *knowledge*.

On the basis of such an assumption, several main components are identified from the Health Care Information System Architecture (HCISA) model: the patient (or subject of care), activity, medical record, resource, authorization, and knowledge components [CEN 1997b].

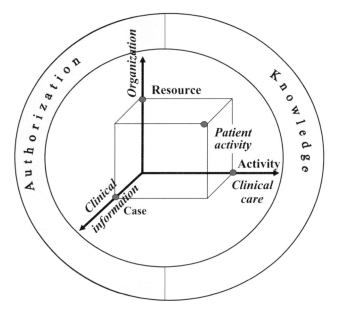

Figure 2.5: Main components of a generic healthcare information system architecture model.

Patient Component

Subjects of care focus on healthcare processes to observe or to change their medical status at an operational level. They include patients and groups of patients. Populations and their needs are sometimes analyzed at the hospital planning level to determine the types of services needed. Other subjects of care are specimens and transplant organs. Specimen may be related to the patient and properties of the specimen may be used in the deduction of the clinical state of a patient. Subjects of care may be interrelated (mother– child, spouse). Relationships may change over time. The main characteristic attributes are

- identification inside and outside the healthcare environment,
- characteristic demographic attributes, and
- location in the healthcare organization.

The patient component (or subject of care component in the HISA model) provides services to client applications to maintain all demographic and administrative data regarding patients (or subjects of care).

Activity Component

The activity component is one of the most important components in achieving the integration of the patients' health care process. Hence the activity component reflects and supports the medical organization as a whole. The activity component governs the flow of work and information between the various healthcare actors based on the output of the scheduling engine (as part of the resource component described below). The activity component is the basis for *provider order entry* (POE) systems. Many argue that the most important long-term benefit of POE results from the integration of clinical decision support systems into the order-entry process [McDonald 1976, Pryor 1990] coupled with a hospital-wide resource scheduling system and with an electronic health record (EHR).

The impact of clinical evidence on clinical practice by means of the creation of clinical protocols represents a major technical challenge and a promising opportunity in the field of medical informatics. In this sense, the activity component is a fundamental element. As is often the case in medical informatics, a system succeeds only if it can seamlessly integrate with other systems. For example one must provide features to take into account, as much as possible, the context in which a protocol will be used.

An activity may be elementary, composite, or repetitive. The establishment of a composite or repetitive activities implies the establishment of the corresponding constituent elementary activities. A drug treatment regimen is an example of a *repetitive* activity. A clinical care pathway that does not involve branching could be specified as a *composite* activity.

Medical activities carried out on behalf of the patient (subject of care) can be classified into two groups:

• Activities that provide information on the healthcare status of the patient. This information can be a quantitative result, a descriptive result, or a combination of both.
• Activities that attempt to change or maintain the health status of the patient.

When an activity is executed, various medical data may be generated as part of the electronic health record. This information may be structured according to the type of activity or the role of the performing healthcare agents.

Resource Management Component

Resource-oriented services provide users with information and functions related to resource availability and allocation. The most important role of the resource component is to solve resource allocation (people, medical devices, tasks, and so on.) and scheduling problems in a tightly constrained environment. Solving these problems is essential, and an important medical and organizational aim in many healthcare organizations in order to operate in an ever more cost-efficient way. Reduced budgets foster the importance of hospital-wide scheduling systems to provide better service to patients while improving resource utilization and increasing staff productivity. State-of-the-art scheduling systems are not designed for a particular service but must be able to span various medical systems and functions involving enterprise-wide thinking as opposed to departmental thinking. These systems use the following components: patient, activity, and resource.

From the point of view of use, resources are classified into active and passive (or consumable) resources. *Active resources* or agents are necessary to perform actions relevant to the provision of health care. Agents are abstractions of human beings involved in the direct or indirect use of healthcare information systems. An agent can be a person, a group of persons, or an institution: physicians, nurses, administrators, and so on. Different roles can be assigned to agents in performing their task according to the group to which they belong and their corresponding security profile.

Passive or consumable resources include medical equipment associated with a location for which scheduling is needed or materials that are used in the process of providing medical care: drugs, disposables, and so on. The utilization of each resource has its specific cost, depending on the resource involved and on the type of activity performed.

Health Record Component

Continuity of care requires a cooperative environment between autonomous complementary health services in terms of data and functionalities. This component offers tools for storing patient data generated during the performance of medical activities such as observational data (physical examination, results from tests) or therapeutic data (medication administered, surgery performed, actions planned). Besides storage, it also enables the display of comprehensive patient data as abstracted information of how (recorded by different staff members), when (different contexts), or where the data were entered. These information sources may exist in separate autonomous systems.

For example, the patient's vital signs can be recorded on three different occasions (by a physician as part of an outpatient visit, by administrative staff as part of the admission procedure, and by a nurse as part of the patient's care plan) in three different forms. The *electronic healthcare record* (EHCR) or more broadly the *electronic health record* (EHR) has to be capable of locating basic patient data captured in the different environments and integrating it into a single view.

Queries are based on the structure defined in the event taxonomy, which are described through the use of metadata. Hence each data set, form, or display used at the application level is broken down into its elementary record item complexes and record items (see chapter 6). The user is not limited to one approach to entering the clinical encounter, and the generic user interface must support a number of data entry facilities. For retrieval, domain-specific queries depending on the application domain are user-configurable.

The EHR is made up of a number of events described by clinical statements. Clinical statements are expressed by means of *record items* (RI) and *record item complexes* in the *Electronic Healthcare Record Architecture* (EHCRA) prestandard of the European standardization committee (CEN/TC251) [CEN 1995, CEN 2000]. Clinical information is documented with additional contextual information and qualifiers. Through the aggregation of record items, each event represents a compound clinical concept at one location at one time. Events correspond in GEHR with the notion of transaction and in SYNAPSES/SYNEX with the comRIC class derived from the record item complex class [Grimson 1998].

The patient data repository is centralized logically but can be physically distributed over several network nodes. This type of architecture offers many advantages: by isolating the patient data repository from multiple services it offers openness and independence.

EHRs grow in size and complexity. Hence, a browser within a *clinical workstation* (CWS) must assist healthcare users to explore the EHR, generate customized overviews, and retrieve detailed information relevant to a particular aspect of care delivery at an appropriate level of granularity. Events are defined by or linked to one or more computer screen forms. Events allow navigation in large EHRs. Also headings, which group a number of similar kinds of record entries with a common subject, can be defined.

Authorization Component

Appropriate security and authentication policies are critical in the healthcare domain. Customizing the presentation layer, access privileges to data and functions are acquired at log-in time from the authorization component that stores information about users, user groups, accessible functions in accordance with the user roles, patient profiles (e.g., employee, VIP), and the ongoing medical activities, equipment localization and usage patterns.

The authorization component contains the profile of each type of agent within the information system authorized to perform various activities and having access to various types of information. Agents are human beings involved in the healthcare process, parts of the organization (medical service), software artifacts, or devices. Profiles are defined according to criteria established in the hospital, depending on the national and regional regulations of the country and based on local rules and on characteristics of the individual activities and data.

Knowledge Management Component

Knowledge can currently be found in many different formats and locations, such as paper and electronic documents, but only a small part is structured in computerized knowledge bases. The knowledge management component plays a key role in clinical information systems. First it assures that certain levels of standards are met by applying intelligent coaching features on top of existing systems (e.g., POE). On the other hand it lets applications from multiple satellite systems coexist by mapping terms or codes used in various applications into a common representation before being piped to the longitudinal patient record.

The knowledge component consists of several subcomponents (or components): the terminology component, the knowledge sources (e.g., in the form of business rules), and the inference engine(s). The *terminology component* handles different types of medical concepts that can be structured in a semantic network of terms constituting the *ontology* of the domain. This component is essential to build up flexible and evolving EHR systems as well as to guarantee semantic integration of the various components.

Multiple formalisms have been proposed to structure *knowledge sources*, including frames, rules, and more complex logical modules described in Chapter 7. Inference engines apply structured knowledge to facts to generate new information or knowledge..

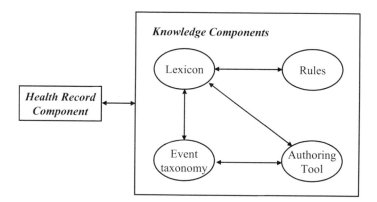

Figure 2.6: Knowledge components accessed by the health record component.

Most components have a strong relationship with the knowledge component that forms the underlying basis for medical decision support systems and verifies the suitability of certain actions. Following are examples of conditions or actions for which decision rules might be useful:

- Prescribe orders that are compatible with the patient's sex, age or condition?

- Check that the patient is available at the time an action is to be carried out.

- Check that the hospital resources (staff, equipment) are available to perform an action at the time requested.

- Do not order tests that have already been ordered.

- Search if a drug contra indicated.
- Avoid ordering a CT scan after a recent barium study.

Figure 2.6 illustrates the interactions between the medical record and the knowledge components. Building an EHR needs access to a lexicon covering a hierarchy of concepts and their semantic links, an events taxonomy, a business rule base, and an authoring component or form editor. The authoring component generates the presentation layer, has access to the lexicon and rules, and enables the creation of the content for import into the EHR.

When a medical event (act, physical examination, history) has to be created, the system searches for the corresponding concept in the lexicon. Through a mapping mechanism, all subsequent lexical items linked to the root concept are mapped dynamically to form a template and presented to the user. The medical record component validates and checks incoming data against the rules defined in the rules engine.

Application Domain

A healthcare organization can be defined as an established organization that carries out specific functions related to healthcare delivery or research in life sciences (Figure 2.7). An organization is the result of unification for a common purpose or function.

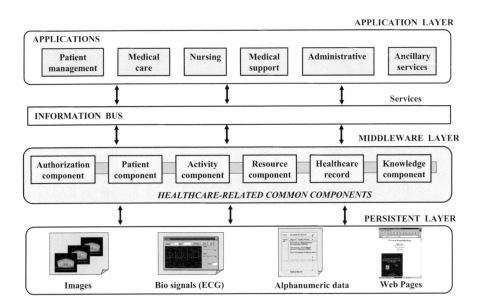

Figure 2.7: A three-layer architecture covering the application domain (clients), business objects, generic services, and a persistent layer (data servers).

Based on the user profiles, a healthcare information system may be clustered in homogeneous groups of activities and data. Several functional healthcare domains, focusing on both inpatients and outpatients, may be identified in a healthcare information system.

- *Patient management.* The patient management area clusters those activities related to the *identification, registration* (admission), and *tracking* of a patient in the healthcare center, and the communication of data with other institutions on a national or international level for statistical purposes. Such activities may operate both at an enterprise level, for the whole healthcare institution, or at the level of an organizational unit.

- *Medical care.* The medical care area clusters activities directly related to prevention, diagnosis, treatment, and follow-up of patients performed by physicians. It accesses records and maintains medical patient data.

- *Medical support.* The aim of this area is the delivery of a set of diagnostic services or treatments on behalf of other healthcare actors in relation to the patient's medical care plan. It aims to increase the information about the patient's health status or improve it. Medical support is composed of several different units such as functional laboratories (laboratories/services devoted to in vivo or in vitro examinations, for diagnostic or therapeutic purposes, ECG, EEG, and so on), imaging services, pharmacy, and social services.

- *Nursing.* The nursing area specifies all activities performed by nurses to support

  - Patients in their daily activities and contribute to their health or recovery.

  - Nurses to maintain their care plans and patient records,

  - Physicians and other clinical professionals in carrying out the medical care plan.

  Nursing activities can be classified in the following main specific classes: ward unit, emergency, recovery, ambulatory care, one-day clinic, and home care.

- *Ancillary services.* The ancillary service area includes activities that are not directly related to the clinical care of the patient but are necessary to facilitate healthcare production. The main functional units are information services, domestic and hotel services, food and diet management, laundry, technical services, and materials management.

- *Administration and management.* This area groups, for strategic and operational purposes, all activities necessary to support policy making, planning, implementation, monitoring, and evaluating the overall functioning of the hospital. The activities are of two types: strategic (planning, acquisition) and operational (financial, organizational, and personnel) management.

Technical Infrastructure

The technical infrastructure concerns the networking environment, persistent storage servers, and other hardware environments. The technical infrastructure must offer a sufficient quality of service in terms of network bandwidth, performance, and availability. The location of a particular service in a layer is not final and may be transferred between layers in the future, depending on the technology.

The global architectural framework is a marriage of business object technology and *N*-tier client/server architectures (Figure 2.8). A 2-tier fat server architecture places more functions on the server side [Orfali 1999]. A 2-tier fat client architectures does the reverse. An *N*-tier architecture divides software processing into *N* cooperative layers. In a 3-tier architecture, the user interface is commonly in the first tier, the databases in the third tier and the application logic in the middle-tier.

	2-tier fat server architecture	2-tier fat client architecture	3-tier client/server architecture
	By performing processing in the database, thick-database architectures can improve performance over fat clients.	Although useful for screen-intensive applications, thick-client architectures don't scale well.	3-tier architectures scale better than fat clients, but they still have to remove data from a database in order to work on it.
Pro	• Has low client-management requirements. • Keeps data manipulation in database for fast performance.	• Offloads processing from central database computer. • Enables users to manipulate data how they want.	• Offloads processing from central database computer. • Has low client-management requirements. • Scales well.
Con	• Can pose a problem for load balancing.	• Increases client-management requirements. • Increases network traffic.	• Possibility of poor performance as data is removed from database.

Figure 2.8: Client/server architectures.

It is helpful to notice the symmetry between user interfaces and databases. Both user interfaces and databases represent views on the model in the MVC paradigm. Indeed, user interfaces (= view) give and receive information from applications, while databases (= another view) communicate in the same way with applications. Changes in the application or database layer have minor effects on the business model.

There are basically three major approaches to object persistence [Stonebraker 1999] solving the so-called impedance mismatch:

- *Middleware-based approach.* Objects are supported in a middleware layer enveloping the DBMS, and the object behavior is called in a different address space using a request broker mechanism (e.g., Oracle 8, Sybase, and Microsoft approach). Other types of commercial systems are Persistence Subtleware/SQL, Gemstone/Gateway, and ObjectStore/Gateway.
- *Object-relational (ORDBMS) approach.* Existing RDBMS are enhanced with an OO-layer serving object simulation. Data processing and management are integrated in a single RDBMS engine (e.g., the IBM and Informix approaches). The SQL standard has been extended to become part of the SQL3 standard.
- *Object-oriented DBMS (OODBMS)* add persistence support to objects in an OO-programming language (e.g., Gemstone, Versant, Objectstore, Ontos, and so on) [Strinvasin 1997].

As the demand for OO-DBMS rises and RDBMS still remains in the mainstream, the middleware-based approach to object persistence, in the absence of approaches (2) and (3), is the most popular. The application (business) servers situated in the middleware do not persistently store the data. Rather, they incorporate the business model controlling the application logic. Hence back-end software artifacts (departmental systems, repositories) may be altered, upgraded, and/or replaced without impacting the CIS functionality (as long as the new/upgraded systems properly register the objects they replace). Likewise, the front-end system (clinical views of the CWS) may be altered from central locations (domain servers) without affecting the back-end systems and without requiring modification of the viewing stations.

The data access subsystem maps information from relational tables into business objects and vice versa. As the number of database connections is limited, a 3-tier architecture circumvents this restriction through multiplexing, a process defined in the literature as database funneling.

Summary and Conclusions

In earlier software development approaches, the emphasis was on data integration, which gave rise to data warehouses. Today the emphasis is on application integration. Yesterday, data was centralized and static. Today data have become distributed and dynamic, requiring software that not only responds to users' requests but also anticipates the medical user in the information overload.

Component frameworks—built on a strong underlying conceptual and technological layer and openness — are the hallmarks of medical informatics today.

Common object request brokers (CORBA), DCOM, and *N*-tier technologies have become mainstream. Servers located in the middle-tier apply the clinical model and application rules to communicate with so-called thin-client workstations. The architecture harmonizes two opposite forces: the user's requirement for autonomy in locating data and functions as close as possible to the originating medical services and the proper management of data [Van de Velde 1992]. Conversely, there is the more enterprise-driven (centralized) approach motivated by the concern for consolidating data as much as possible into one logical computer-based health record due to the increased complexity, technical (connectivity), and semantic integration challenges intrinsically related to this distributed philosophy. Rather than misuse our creative abilities in "reinventing the wheel" for every project, we must focus on the reusability, maintainability, and interoperability of the core business processes. These assets need to be constructed within an overall architecture that is designed from the top down and that accommodates a high rate of both business and technological changes [Plachy 1998]. The *N*–tier approach, compared with third and fourth generation languages (GL) development environments, provides a richer, more scalable, and more viable application in the long term but at the expense of a lower return on investment due to a steeper learning curve and a less productive environment. Above all one must adhere to a movement away from a technically driven solution toward a more knowledge-driven solution.

Hospital users try to get the most from their information system. The ultimate objective of the development of an integrated reference architecture for a clinical information system must be the provision of an environment for transforming data into useful information regardless of the location and characteristics of the networked information sources. Protecting existing legacy systems while integrating new applications, mapping the future while change is constant and unpredictable technically, and choosing the right vendors when new ones appear are the greatest challenges. It is to be hoped that patients will also experience the benefits of these technological advances [Orphanoudakis 1996].

References

[Booch 1994] Booch G. *Object-Oriented Analysis and Design with Applications, 2nd ed.* Redwood City, Calif.: Benjamin/Cummings, 1994.

[Booch 1999] Booch G, Rumbaugh J, Jacogson I. *The Unified Modeling Language User Guide*. Reading, Massachusetts: Addison-Wesley, 1999.

[Brown 2000] Brown AW. *Large-Scale Component-Based Development.* Upper Saddle River, N.J.: Prentice Hall, 2000.

[Bohrer 1998] Bohrer BA. Architecture of the San Francisco frameworks. *IBM Systems J.* 1998; 37(2):156–169. [http://www. almaden.ibm.com/journal/].

[CEN 1995] CEN/TC251. *PrENV 12265. Electronic Healthcare Record Architecture*. July 1995. [http://www.centx251.org].

[CEN 1997] CEN/TC251. *PrENV 12967-1. Healthcare Information System Architecture Part 1 (HISA)—Healthcare Middleware Layer*. March 1997. [http://www.centx251.org].

[CEN 2000] CEN/TC251. *PrENV 13606-1. Electronic Healtcare Record Communication*. May 2000. [http://www.centx251.org].

[Cummins 2002] Cummins FA. *Enterprise Integration—An Architecture for Enterprise Application and Systems Integration*. New York: John Wiley & Sons, 2002.

[Graham 1995] Graham I. *Migrating to Object Technology*. Reading, Massachusetts: Addison-Wesley, 1995.

[Ferrara 1998] Ferrara FM. The standard "Healthcare Information Systems Architecture" and the DHE middleware. *Int J Med Inf.* 1998; 52 (1-3): 39–51.

[Grimson 1998] Grimson W, Berry D, Grimson J, Stephens G, Felton E, Given P, O'Moore R. Federated healthcare record server—the Synapses Paradigm. *Int J Med Inf.* 1998; 52 (1–3): 3–27.

[Hammond 1994] Hammond WE. The role of standards in creating a health information infrastructure. *Int J Biomed Comput.* 1994; 34: 29–44.

[Herzum 2000] Herzum P, Sims O. *Business Component Factory—A Comprehensive Overview of Component-Based Development for the Enterprise*. New York: John Wiley & Sons, 2000.

[IBM 1998] IBM. San Francisco Team. *San Francisco Business Process, Components. A Technical Introduction*. 1998.

[IMG 1992] Information Management Group. *The Cosmos Project*. NHS Information Management Centre. 1992; Version 2.0; vol. 1–2.

[Jacobson 1992] Jacobson I. *Object-Oriented Software Engineering: A Use Case Driven Approach*. Wokingham, England: Addison-Wesley, 1992.

[Leisch 1997] Leisch E, Sartzetakis S, Tsiknakis M, Orphanoudakis SC. A framework for the integration of distributed autonomous healthcare information systems. *J Med Informatics*. 1997; 22(4): 325–335.

[Linthicum 1999] Linthicum DS. Java and ActiveX find transactionality. Update your traditional computing. *Components Strategies*. 1999; 1(7): 46–50.

[McDonald 1976] McDonald CJ. Protocol-based computer reminders, the quality of care and the non perfectibility of man. *N Engl J Med.* 1976; 295(24): 1351–1355.

[Monday 1998] Monday P, Rubin B. Business process components and infrastructure. *Java Report*. 1998; 3 (3): 51–58.

[OMG 1997] Object Management Group. Common Business Objects. White paper. December 4, 1997. [www.omg.org, document bom/97-12-04].

[Orphanoudakis 1996] Orphanoudakis SC, Kaldoudi E, Tsiknakis M. Technological advances in teleradiology. *Eur J Radiol.* 1996; 22(3): 205–217.

[Orfali 1997] Orfali R, Harkey D. *Instant CORBA*. New York: John Wiley & Sons, 1997.

[Orfali 1999] Orfali R, Harkey D, Edwards J. *Client/Server Survival Guide, 3rd Edition*. New York: John Wiley & Sons, 1999.

[Plachy 1998] Plachy EC, Hausler PA. Enterprise Solutions Structure. *IBM Systems J.* 1998; 38(1).

[Pryor 1990] Pryor TA, Dupont R, Clay J. A MLM based order entry systems. *Proc 14th Annual Symp Comput Appl Med Care.* 1990; 579–83.

[RICHE 1992] Riche Consortium. *RICHE ESPRIT project.* Final Report. November 30, 1992.

[Rumbaugh 1991] Rumbaugh J, Blaha M, Premerlani W, Eddy F, Lorensen W. *Object-Oriented Modeling and Design*. Upper Saddle River, NJ. Prentice Hall, 1991.

[Stonebraker 1999] Stonebraker M, Brown P. *Objects in Middleware: How bad can it be?* April 15, 1999. [http://www.itpapers.com/].

[Strinvasin 1997] Strinvasin, Chang DT. Object Persistence in object-oriented applications. *IBM Systems J.* 1997; 1(36): 66–87.

[Tsiknakis 1997] Tsiknakis M, Chronaki CE, Kapidakis S, Nikolaou C, Orphanoudakis SC. An integrated architecture for the provision of health telematic services based on digital library technologies. *Int J Digit Libr.* 1997 (3): 257–77.

[Usoft 1998] Usoft. *Automation: A Proven Approach and Software Technology to Implement Computing Applications*. White paper 1998.

[Van de Velde 1992] Van de Velde R. *Hospital Information Systems—The next generation*. Heidelberg: Springer-Verlag, 1992.

[Van de Velde 1997] Van de Velde R. *Alternative Proposal for a Healthcare Information System Architecture*. Technical report PT013. Barcelona, Spain: PT013 workgroup. May 10–13, 1997.

[Wilson 1999] Wilson C. Application architectures with enterprise Java-Beans. *Component Strategies.* 1999; 2(2): 25–34.

3

Frameworks: A Collaboration of Objects

Observe, however, that of man's whole terrestrial possessions and attainments, unspeakably the noblest are his symbols.

—Thomas Carlyle

The most important objective of medicine today is to *share* and *reuse* medical information and knowledge. To exchange and compare data and knowledge between various heterogeneous, often incompatible medical systems (information component systems, healthcare actors, etc.), people need a common channel over which to communicate and a common view of the domain of discourse to understand one another.

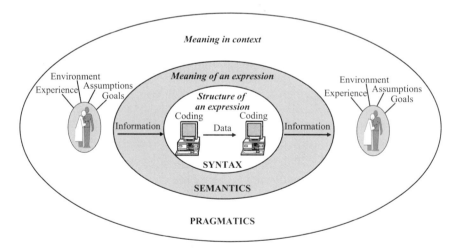

Figure 3.1: Exchange of messages between two independent systems.

Sharing and communicating information between healthcare agents is feasible only if one agrees on the format, content, structure, and meaning of the exchanged messages (Figure 3.1). Therefore, it is important that the sender and receiver of information use the same language to express very precisely the many details of information in medicine [Rossi 1994, Degoulet 1999].

This chapter provides an overview of different standardized approaches to message exchange. Exchanges modalities are then considered in a situation of collaboration between a set of interrelated components.

Dimensions in Communications

Communication and collaboration between agents can be looked at from the infrastructure or applicative point of view.

Infrastructure Level

The infrastructure/computational level corresponds to the message exchange format that deals with the communication and transport protocols used and to the low-level communication layers. Referring to the OSI (Open System Interconnection) model of ISO (International Standard Organization), they correspond to layers 1 (Physical) to 6 (Presentation). On the lowest level we define the channels (network connections, satellite links, telephones, ...) and services to carry and accomplish the communication.

Applicative Level

The applicative level corresponds to the content of the message and deals with the syntax, semantic, and pragmatic level. In terms of the OSI model it corresponds to layer 7 (Application).

The syntax level *(format)* describes the rules that govern how strings, characters, and words may be combined to define data messages and control information (e.g., data types, structures, and relationships) and requires that applications agree on a common format for the data. These rules describe messages used to interchange information between healthcare information systems and define information that attributes the sequence and physical representation of the messages.

The semantic level (*meaning*) conveys the meaning of the message and requires agreement on a common understanding for the data. An external terminology system representing medical concepts explains the meaning. Most healthcare organizations identify their data by means of their internal (and idiosyncratic) code values. As a result, receiving systems often cannot fully understand these data unless they share the sender's codes (if they receive results from multiple organizations, this is practically impossible). Although sufficient technology is available today, one item that has generally been missing, an item essential to the vision of information sharing, exchange, and reuse between clinicians and between the clinician and the computer, is something to bond all the different components of a heterogeneous medical world together. That bonding material or "glue" [Hausam 1996] is a standardized clinical vocabulary (also known as a controlled medical terminology or several other variations of the same name). A standardized clinical vocabulary provides a means of accurately, clearly, and reliably communicating medical information [Cimino 2001].

The pragmatic level (*contextual information*) defines information and knowledge about the context of communication message production. With the semantic level, the pragmatic level supports part of the meaning of a communication message.

Complexity and difficulties arise from the lowest to the highest level of communication. However, the higher one climbs, the more difficult it becomes to agree on a common understanding of the elements communicated.

Communication Standards

This section aims to provides an overview of the major existing and emerging healthcare information standards in a bottom-up fashion from the syntax to the pragmatic level (Figure 3.2). A standard is a collection of specifications that has been endorsed by a group. In the last two decades, several organizations have proposed data exchange standards. Most standards are unfortunately defined at the syntax level.

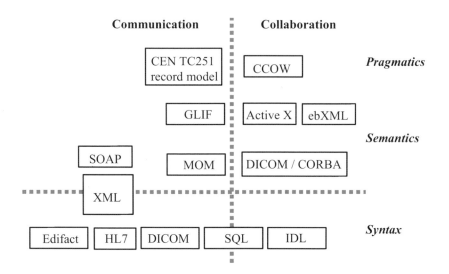

Figure 3.2: Overview of various existing standards focusing on the communication between agents.

Communication at the Syntax Level

Generic standards such as ASN.1, EDIFACT, XML or SOAP are domain-independent. Standards dedicated to the healthcare domain have also been proposed in the last two decades (e.g., HL7, DICOM, MIB). The current trend is now to specialize a generic standard such as XML to cover the specific aspects of a domain.

ASN.1

Abstract Syntax Notation One is a language that defines how data are sent over a network across dissimilar communication systems. It provides a common syntax defined in OSI layer 6 so that different systems can understand each other's data structures. ASN.1 uses a set of Basic Encoding Rules (BERs) based on a list of data types and their assigned numbers in ASN.1 notation.

EDIFACT

EDIFACT (Electronic Data Interchange For Administration Commerce and Transport) is an ISO standard for electronic data interchange (EDI) that was proposed to supersede both X12 and TRADACOMS as the worldwide standard.

XML

XML (Extensible Mark-up Language) is gaining popularity [Moshfeghi 1999] and is largely used in messaging. XML incorporates meta data and uses tags to define the overall structure and relationships between types of text and data. This is done in the DTD (Document Type Definition). XML can deliver structured data to the desktop, compute the data via the object model, apply formatting rules to the data with the XSL (eXtensible Stylesheet Language) environment, and present the data in HTML (HyperText Markup Language).

It is also important to mention the possibilities of XML as a distributed data format compared with broker systems such as CORBA and COM. Before being implemented, both technologies have to be studied in the context in which they will be used. XML is better at handling huge sets of text data and diagram versioning. As a result, it is used to manage document and manipulate stream-based data. CORBA provides a distributed message framework and supports machine-readable non text data [Deadman 1999].

Data contained in various heterogeneous autonomous medical systems (cardiology, neurology, nephrology, etc.) can be sent on a regular basis as well-formed XML messages to a middle-tier server. The beauty and power of XML is that it separates the presentation (displaying XML-based data in HTML using XSL) from the data and provides the possibility of describing the entire scope of medical information through a universal method in XML format, allowing the seamless integration of data from diverse sources. This fetch mechanism can be initiated through a workflow component that retrieves all the data from diverse satellite systems on a regular basis. As those systems may contain identical semantic information in various syntactical forms, on-the-fly conversion (mediation mechanism) is needed. Data in XML format are parsed, manipulated, and stored in the appropriate business component. Sometimes data must be converted into XML in the middle tier. XML may be accompanied with DTDs to validate the data when the receiving application does not have a built-in description of the incoming data.

HL7

A consortium of suppliers (system vendors) and users produced the HL7 specification (Figure 3.3). Health Level 7 (HL7) refers to the highest level of the OSI reference model. However, HL7 is not fully compliant with the OSI framework. The objective was the formatting and exchanging of data between health care institutions, particularly hospitals, and between different computer systems within hospitals, with emphasis on patient administration (patient registration, admission, discharge and transfer), patient orders, and results from ancillary services (laboratories, pharmacy, diet, and radiology image studies), supplier orders, insurance, and financial (charging and paying) information. The data structures are limited to text, with one extension to support a formatted screen display in response to a query.

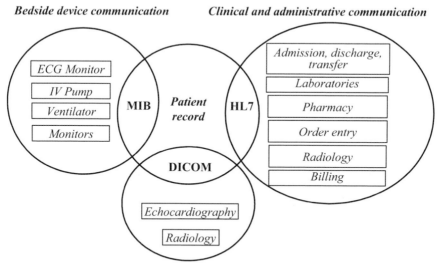

Figure 3.3: Standards dealing with data exchange in a healthcare setting: HL7, MIB, and DICOM.

Exchange of clinical data, such as patient orders and results, is closely harmonized with the ASTM E1238 standard. HL7 has incorporated E1238 as a subset within the laboratory results message format. Recently, the HL7 and

ASTM E1238 committees have been working very closely, and further developments are expected to result in the convergence of the two specifications.

Task forces in HL7 are currently developing prototype transactions with new object-oriented technologies such as CORBA and Microsoft's ActiveX objects and transactions for exchanging information about appointment scheduling, problem lists, clinical trial enrollments, patient permissions, voice dictations, advanced directives, and electro-physiological signals.

Implementation of the HL7 standard is not straightforward, but the advantages gained over time are worthwhile. For instance, within HL7 there is no model for conformance and, although it leaves room for interpretation to give each user and vendor the freedom to insert his or her proper needs, each implementation has to be studied in detail. The HL7 organization provides for interpretative flexibility for the following reasons:

- Different organizations have different information needs (e.g., specific demographic country-dependent data.
- Specific design features should not be implied.
- Optional features are accepted.

DICOM ACR/NEMA

The American College of Radiology (ACR) and the National Electrical Manufacturers Association (NEMA) compiled a standard for the formatting, communication, and storage of digital images and associated data (HIS/RIS information) for devices of different suppliers such as computed tomography, magnetic resonance imaging, nuclear medicine, ultrasounds or video capture. DICOM has two components: image format standardization and image communications protocols.

Image format standard allows image data compatibility among various vendors. Image communications protocols permit the exchange of radiologic images and other medical information between computers [George 1999]. It also supports the connection of networked printers, such as laser imagers (cameras). The standard gives substance to layers 1 to 7 of the OSI reference model, but is not fully compatible with it.

DICOM is a large and complex standard and no products implement the entire standard. Specific requirements need to be defined for each application. Beyond device conformance, it is very important to determine if the usability of the device in the specific DICOM environment will meet the clinical needs. Therefore, it is advisable to clearly understand what vendors mean when they say their products are "DICOM conformant" and ensure that different products are able to work together.

The DICOM standard incorporates an object-oriented data model and provides full networking capability. It also includes a RIS/HIS-interface.

MIB

Wide ranges of instruments used in hospitals lack a common means for data acquisition and do not even offer computer-addressable interfaces. The Medical Information Bus (MIB), the IEEE 1073 standard for medical device communications, was designed to solve the problem of communication between a myriad of sophisticated medical devices from different manufacturers with a common interface. Those devices are found in an acute-care environment such the intensive care unit (ICU) or operating room, where safety, reliability, and ease-of-use requirements need to be met. In such environments, the bedside configuration dependent on the patient's condition constantly changes over time, requiring that instruments be disconnected and reconnected. Hence, MIB associates devices with a specific patient, no matter where the patient is located, and provides clinicians with *dynamic reconfiguration facilities*. IEEE 1073 is backed by a number of suppliers of medical instruments and organizations.

From the hardware viewpoint, the MIB uses a polled twisted-pair network running at 9600 bauds. A bus can have up to 255 instruments attached. Each device is identified by an ID code that identifies each device and a common descriptor for each class of machine (i.e., describing the functions and parameters it registers). The MIB automatically detects whether devices are connected or disconnected.

The MIB can be applied to the following instruments:

- noninvasive and invasive measurement instruments (pulse rate, atrial and ventricular blood pressure),
- fluid delivery intravenous (IV) pumps and fluid collection devices (chest drainage, urine output), and
- respiratory instruments (ventilators).

The MIB operates under a master–slave communication protocol. From the software viewpoint, the master–slave communication protocol is a subset of the highly reliable synchronous data link control (SDLC) protocol [Gardner 1986].

The central device or master communication controller (MCC) polls all the medical instruments and recognizes when devices are present or not on the network. A special-purpose medical device language (MDL) has been proposed for message interchange. The slave is the interface between the bedside instrument and the MIB and is called the device communications controller (DCC). An overview of monitoring parameters and biosignals as a basis for continuous or intermittent patient monitoring can be found in [Van de Velde 1992].

Since some of the MIB layers are not yet approved, its current use is limited. With just physical layers available in its current version, it is ineffective in addressing the problem of device integration. As a result, compatible acquisition software is necessary to ensure the communication between the many sophisticated data medical devices in the acute-care environment.

Communication at the Semantic Level

LOINC

To facilitate the exchange of clinical laboratory data, LOINC (Logical Observation Identifiers, Names, and Codes) [Bakken 2000] provides a set of universal names and ID codes for identifying laboratory and clinical findings. Unlike other coding systems, this one does not require a license fee. The files that constitute the codes, user manual, and other parts of the offering can be downloaded.

Currently, many laboratories are using ASTM 1238-94 or its sister standard, HL7, to send laboratory results electronically from producer laboratories to clinical care systems in hospitals.

If laboratories all used the LOINC codes to identify their results in data transmissions, the compatibility problem would be alleviated. The receiving system with LOINC codes in its master vocabulary file would be able to understand and properly file HL7 results messages that also use the LOINC code.

GALEN and the GRAIL Language

GALEN (Generalized Architecture for Languages, Encyclopaedias and Nomenclatures in medicine) is an European Union funded AIM project (A2012) aiming to develop the foundations for the next generation of computer-based multilingual coding systems for medicine [Rector 1998, Rogers 2001]. The project has developed a scheme in which key medical concepts can be represented. The medical concepts represented using this scheme must be accessible and manipulable by computers. The representation scheme is known as GRAIL (GALEN Representation And Integration Language). The model becomes language- and application-independent when using GRAIL, known as the CORE (COmmon REference) model.

GALEN encapsulates the knowledge in the CORE model in software servers (known as terminology servers) that access the model for applications and provide a standard interface to it. The terminology servers are intended to support the requirements of individual applications for multilingual clinical terminology, to mediate between existing systems, and to facilitate the development of new systems.

KIF

KIF (Knowledge Interchange Format) is a very expressive language for the interchange of knowledge. It has declarative semantics (i.e., the meaning of expressions can be understood without using an interpreter). It is logically comprehensive in that it provides tools for the expression of arbitrary sentences in the first-order predicate calculus, for the definition of objects, functions, and relations, the representation of metaknowledge, and the declaration of nonmonotonic reasoning rules [Finin 1999].

Communication at the Pragmatic Level

The Pragmatic Component of the CENT TC251 Patient Record Model

The European Healthcare Record Architecture (EHCRA) defines the basic architectural principles for representing the content and structure of all electronic healthcare records [CEN 2000]. It facilitates deciding what to store and in which format. It supports a common understanding of the variable content and format of records. It is neither a system specification nor a standardized healthcare record. It provides the foundation for a standard reference architecture for the interchange of electronic healthcare records (in whole or part) between electronic healthcare record systems.

The scope is deliberately limited in four ways:

1. Because this standard is in the information domain and not in the knowledge domain, it does not determine or constrain the structure of clinical knowledge.
2. As an architecture for the electronic healthcare record, it does not apply to

   a. electronic healthcare system architecture or design;

   b. healthcare domain information models;

   c. syntaxes for the presentation or identification of information in a record; or

   d. specifications for the representation of information elements (e.g., images, sound, structured text) in the electronic healthcare record.
3. It does not specify an interchange format or how to perform interchange of electronic healthcare records.
4. It represents a foundation standard and requires further standards.

Collaboration Between Objects

Collaboration via the WWW

The World Wide Web (WWW), initiated as a great platform for electronic publishing, has opened new opportunities for building client interfaces to access Internet and Intranet Servers and has evolved into a planetary operating system [Udell 1996]. Applications are not confined to stand-alone computers. They run on all kinds of processors and they exchange and share data with computers distributed on wide-area networks. Web-smart, platform-independent applications are gradually used more and more for software development. This could pave the way for a new interaction metaphor in the man–machine interface for tomorrow's clinical workstation: the hypertext metaphor that visualizes data as a network of linked parts.

HTTP (HyperText Transfer Protocol) can be used as an invocation mechanism to access documents from a document server (HTTPd) or from file (database) servers converting data into documents through the use of Common Gateway Interface (CGI) scripts for SQL databases. One way to create Web pages with active content for relatively simple components is to embed executable scripts in HTML-defined Web pages (Java script, VB script).

HTML pages can be expanded, unlike an applet which is designed to run within a Web page in a browser. A servlet is designed to run on a Web server with servlets. Like an applet, a servlet is a small Java application.

Request Brokers

Objects are the unit of distribution. Communication is provided through a central message-passing medium or broker. A broker is just an object-oriented (OO) mechanism to allow methods to be called on remote objects and is responsible for the transportation of calls from the client application to the target object and the transportation of results. To avoid the client having to know the location of a server object, the broker implements a repository mechanism.

The use of a central message broker shields the user from having to know the physical locations of the objects. CORBA, Microsoft's DCOM, and SUN's Remote Method Invocation (RMI), are mechanisms for one object to call another without regard to its physical location.

CORBA, the Common Object Request Broker Architecture, is currently the most mature middleware architecture for distributed object-oriented applications in heterogeneous environments. In contrast, RMI and DCOM operate in a homogeneous environment. Concepts such as proxies allow accessing remote objects transparently. Additional services that cover a broad spectrum of needs—known as object services (the transactional processing of method calls, the persistent storage of objects, and the availability of security mechanisms, as well as access to distributed objects using a name service)—are required.

The Object Request Broker (ORB) is the heart of the CORBA architecture and supports operations on all the declared objects. Objects may be defined at various levels of granularity. For instance, patient demographics might be defined as an accessible object (through a patient identifier), whereas at a broader level a laboratory report could be defined as a single object.

The CORBA Interface Definition Language (IDL) defines the objects that can be accessed through the ORB. The IDL language is implemented by mapping on available programming languages. CORBA explicitly defines these mappings on C++ and Java.

IIOP (Internet Inter-ORB Protocol) defines the transport service for all remote communications. Other services have been defined within the CORBA environment, but IIOP is the recommended service. Its level is very similar to the HTTP Web protocol.

All names in CORBA are related to a particular context and the naming service operates and maintains that relationship. Names are therefore independent of language, hardware environment and location. The service includes creating, removing and listing objects, together with providing the binding information when requested.

An object reference is established for every name. This object reference is a pointer to the location of the object. A name is unique in a CORBA domain. Most implementations have a single master file that contains the names directory.

The life cycle service creates, deletes, copies, and moves distributed objects in multiple locations. The event service provides a message broadcast service.

If clients and servers were to communicate directly with the broker, then they would have to use a fixed protocol. For this reason two additional layers of indirection are necessary. For every class to be referenced, two special classes must be used: the *proxy* (stub) and the *skeleton*. The proxy is an object that has the same interface as the remote object. Each object is associated with one specific object server. Messages sent to the proxies are marshalled to the remote system, call the same methods on the remote object and return the result.

The proxy acts just like client for the server object being called. Communications (or interactions) over network boundaries, with remote objects residing on object servers, are forwarded automatically by local proxy objects that act as a surrogate (local representative or stand-in) for remote objects. Interactions (or services that an object client may invoke) between objects are enabled by a specific interface, defined by the OMG's Interface Definition Language (IDL) (compiler), that abstracts the functionalities (or services) provided by each object. Just as DTD in XML provides a feature to share the structure of the tag sets, IDL is within CORBA the language-neutral shared definition of object types [Deadman 1999]. CORBA achieves programming language independence by means of the IDL. Vendors are required to offer interoperability on the basis of TCP/IP. In order to exchange information using TCP/IP, brokers must use the standardized IIOP protocol.

Another issue is to ensure that system performance meets the users' requirements that may be limited by database performance, network bandwidth, and ORB response times. An important consideration during the design of the system is the choice of granularity of the distributed objects on the network. As part of the total transaction time, the response time for transactions over a typical CORBA network lasts an average of 5 milliseconds; therefore, it is essential that a user dialogue not require too many transactions [Orfali 1997]. The overhead of transferring a container of one large object is small compared to the overhead of separately transferring each small object of the set if the entire set is required for viewing.

Downloadable Components

Downloadable components are pieces of software that are fetched for the user (client) only when that specific software (functional) is needed. In the race to build powerful downloadable components, Sun Microsystems and Microsoft are battling each other for domination, with Java cross-platform "applets" and Active-X components/controls respectively. The idea is to keep significant code for the functions on the server and the code for the interface on the client. Hence, the integration of Java applets, Active-X controls, CORBA components, CM components, and WWW documents into a composite application framework remains important. Microsoft has positioned DCOM as a competing standard for CORBA. A key industry development fusing these initiatives together could be OMG's CORBA [O'Brien 1996]. Java is being integrated into the OMG's distributed object model, and other OMG-products (e.g., ORBIX from IONA) further integrate Active-X controls.

OMG CORBAmed Approach

CORBAmed has defined health care system templates (HCST) that are a combination of healthcare modules and their interactions.

Five CORBAmed services that provide a very generic framework for the entire health information infrastructure are defined [Hinchley 1998a, 1998b]. The aim is to improve interoperability in the healthcare industry among healthcare organizations by using CORBA technologies (OMG technology) to standardize interfaces for healthcare objects (Figure 3.4).

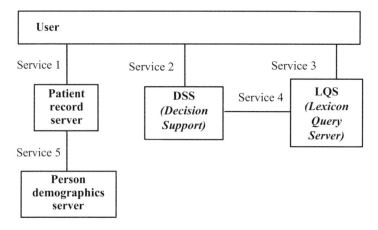

Figure 3.4: The CORBAmed Health Care System Template (CHST).

- Service 1: Patient record inquiries, item entries and updates. Defines a standard method of locating identifiers of individuals and their associated records across facilities and enterprises. This interface must be subject to confidentiality concerns and the right to anonymous care.

- Service 2: Decision support services to the user.
- Service 3: Lexicon query services to the user. Common access to medical terminology resources.
- Service 4: Lexicon query services to the decision support service. Common access to medical terminology resources.
- Service 5: Demographical services related to individuals in the patient record server. Clinical observation retrieval and display. Common interface for the query and display of clinical observations.

CCOW

An excellent example of collaboration between objects that preserves the patient context is found in the Clinical Context Object Workgroup (CCOW) standard. The CCOW standard makes the sharing of healthcare applications in a single visual environment feasible and convenient [Rishel 2000] (Figure 3.5).

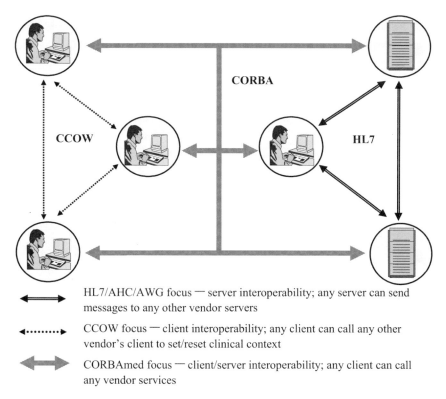

HL7/AHC/AWG focus — server interoperability; any server can send messages to any other vendor servers

CCOW focus — client interoperability; any client can call any other vendor's client to set/reset clinical context

CORBAmed focus — client/server interoperability; any client can call any vendor services

Figure 3.5: Interoperability initiatives at a glance. AHC = ActiveX for health care (Microsoft); AWG = Andover Working Group.

CCOW uses front-end integration to visually synchronize disparate applications. Without achieving plug-and-play integration, CCOW has reduced integration costs and time frames and has helped to facilitate the distributed approach. When each application system had its own users on its own terminals, database synchronization was the primary problem. Today, however, the workstation is a new focal point for visual integration. Visual integration helps to address the transitional challenge faced by CIOs.

CCOW became part of the Health Level Seven Standards Organization and defines a standard that enables the visual integration of independently developed healthcare applications. When visually integrated, these applications work together in ways that the user can see. The patient link capability enables the user to select a patient from any application on a clinical workstation, and have all of the applications automatically "tune in" to the same patient. The user link capability enables a user to sign on to any application on a clinical workstation as the means for securely signing on to all the other applications.

Scenarios in Distributed Environments

There are at least three scenarios available to access various heterogeneous systems. In the traditional approach, access to each system is effected through a separate and appropriate interface (Figure 3.6a).

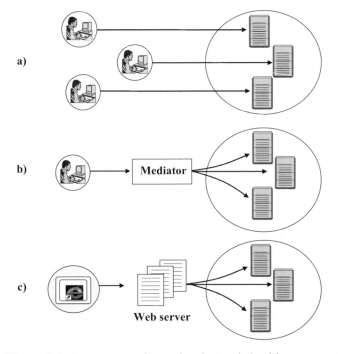

Figure 3.6: Access scenarios to the electronic healthcare record.

In the second approach accesses are effected through a mediator server for which the Synapses project in Europe is one of the first examples (Figure 3.6b) [Grimson 1998, Hinchley 1998b]. In the third approach, the federated access to distributed servers is done through a Web browser with or without a coordination tool (Figure 3.6c). The SynEx project in Europe initiated in July 1998 attempts to provide an open and standard integration platform in which both new and legacy medical applications could easily exchange information. It enables the collaboration of distributed and heterogeneous healthcare records and services, and aims at providing access to hospital information services, to remote sources of medical data and to medical knowledge seamlessly while masking the distribution aspects and the heterogeneity of systems. The SynEx integration platform relies on the DHE (Distributed Healthcare Environment) [Ferrara 1998], a middleware implementation of "HISA" (prENV 12967-1 European Standard Health care Information System Architecture) [CEN 1997]. In the context of the SynEx European project, two software components have been developed by the Medical IT department of Broussais University Hospital in Paris (France): the Pilot and the Mediator components [Xu 2000]. The mediator component is used to manage different connections mechanisms and mainly deal with the syntax and semantics aspects of connections between SynEx components. It provides a generic and flexible way to generate specific mediators. The pilot component manages the workflow of exchanges when several distributed components are involved [Xu 2001].

Summary and Conclusions

Although existing standards and technologies enable us to transmit every bit of information, we should not be distracted from the real challenge, that is how to express healthcare information. G. Schadow stated [McDonald 1997]:

> No interface engine will solve this problem. We must do it. We must standardize the health care information interdisciplinarily and globally. We must provide proper semantics and pragmatics for expressions of health care information for the purpose of communication. Neither SGML nor MIME nor CORBA nor any other technology will help us in doing our homework. The opposite is true: all these fancy technologies have repeatedly distracted our attention towards issues that are secondary. Leaving our homework undone.

References

[Bakken 2000] Bakken S, Cimino JJ, Haskell R, Kukafka R, Matsumoto C, Chan GK, Huff SM. Evaluation of the clinical LOINC (logical observation identifiers, names, and codes) semantic structure as a terminology model for standardized assessment measures. *J Am Med Inform Assoc.* 2000; 7(6): 529–538.

[CEN 1997] CEN/TC251. *PrENV 12967-1. Healthcare Information System Architecture Part 1 (HISA) - Healthcare Middleware Layer.* Brussels: CEN TC251, March 1997. [http://www.centx251.org].

[CEN 2000] CEN/TC251. *PrENV13606-1. Health Informatics - Electronic Healthcare Record Communication.* Brussels: CEN TC251, May 2000. [http://www.centx251.org].

[Cimino 2001] Terminology tools: state of the art and practical lessons. *Meth Inform Med.* 2001; 40(4): 298–306.

[Deadman 1999] Deadman R. XML as a distributed Application Protocol. *Java Report.* 1999; 4(10): 16–21.

[Degoulet 1999] Degoulet P, Fieschi M. *Introduction to Clinical Informatics. Revised Edition.* NewYork: Springer Verlag, 1999.

[Deibel 1999] Deibel SRA. *Introduction to the InterMed Common Guideline Model and Guideline Interchange Format (GLIF)*, 1999. [http://dsg.harvard.edu/public/intermed/glif_overview.html].

[Ferrara 1998] Ferrara FM. The standard "Healthcare Information Systems Architecture" and the DHE middleware. *Int J Med Inf.* 1998; 52 (1-3): 39–51.

[Finin 1999] Finnin T. *UMBC Agent Web maintained at the UMBC Lab for Advanced Information Technology*.1999 [http://www.cs.umbc.edu/kse/].

[Gardner 1986] Gardner RM. Computerized management of intensive care patients. *MD Computing.* 1986; 3 (1): 36–51.

[George 1999] George C, Sun HK, Huang D, Scalzi G. Experiences of healthcare integrated picture archiving and communications systems (PACS). In: *Proc HIMSS.* 1999; 2: 195–210.

[Grimson 1998] Grimson W, Berry D, Grimson J, Stephens G, Felton E, Given P, O'Moore R. Federated healthcare record server - the Synapses Paradigm. *Int J Med Inf.* 1998; 52 (1-3): 3–27.

[Hausam 1996] Hausam RR. *Vocabulary, Coding and Concept Representation.* Florida, Family Physician, 1996; 46(1). [http://www.med.ufl.edy/medinfo//ffp/coding.html, University of Utah].

[Hinchley 1998a] Hinchley A. *Health Informatics Enabling Technologies: CORBA and Microsoft COM/DCOM first draft report TC251,* May 1998.

[Hinchley 1998b] Hinchley A. *Short Strategic Study: Enabling Technologies - COBRA and COM/ DCOM* (Final Report) CEN TC251 N98-108, 1998; pp. 11–23

[McDonald 1997] McDonald CJ, Overhage JM, Dexter P, Takesue B, Suico JG. What is done what is needed, and what is realistic to expert from medical informatics standards. *MIM News.* 1997; 2: 9–14.

[Moshfeghi 1999] Moshfeghi M, de Greef G. XML in a multi-tier Java/CORBA architecture. *IEEE 8th International Workshops on Enabling Technologies: Infrastructure for Collaborative Enterprises.* California: Stanford University,1999.

[O'Brien 1996] O'Brien T. Java/ActiveX rivalry will subside as market pressures forces interoperability. *Object Magazine.* 1996; 6 (6): 18–19.

[Orfali 1997] Orfali R, Harkey D. *Client/Server Programming with Java and CORBA.* New York: John Wiley and Sons, 1997.

[Rector 1998] Rector A, Rossi A, Consorti MF, Zanstra P. Practical development of re-usable terminologies: GALEN-IN-USE and the GALEN Organisation. *Int J Med Inf.* 1998; 48(1-3): 71–84.

[Rishel 2000] Rishel W. *The Clinical Context Object Workgroup: Its Standard and Methods.* White paper, 1998. [http://www.hl7.org/library/Commitees/sigvi/CCOW].

[Rogers 2001] Rogers J, Roberts A, Solomon D, van der Haring E, Wroe C, Zanstra P, Rector A. GALEN ten years on: tasks and supporting tools. *Medinfo* 2001;10 (Pt 1): 256–260.

[Rossi 1994] Rossi Mori A. Co-operative development of a shared ontology for medicine. *CEN/TC251/WG2 IMIA WG 6 - Working Conference.* Geneva, May 29 to June 1, 1994.

[Synapses 2000] *Synapses Synex project.* 2000. http://www.hbroussais.fr/Broussais/InforMed/Genie.

[Udell 1996] Udell J. Your Business Needs the Web. *Byte.* August 1996; 68–80.

[Van de Velde 1992] Van de Velde R. *Hospital Information Systems. The Next Generation.* Berlin: Springer-Verlag, 1992.

[Xu 2000] Xu Y, Sauquet D, Zapletal E, Lemaitre D, Degoulet P. Integration of medical applications: the "mediator service" of the SynEx platform. *Int J Med Inf.* 2000; 58-59: 157–166.

[Xu 2001] Xu Y, D'Alessio L, Jaulent MC, Sauquet D, Spahni S, Degoulet P. Integrating medical applications in an open architecture through generic and reusable components. *Medinfo* 2001; 10 (Pt 1): 63–67.

4

The Patient Component

The *patient component* (subject of care component in the HISA model) is a key component in any healthcare information system that supports clinical, administrative, or epidemiologic activities [CEN 1997]. The patient component is responsible for the correct and permanent identification of a patient in the healthcare organization, the processing (storage and retrieval) of basic patient data, and the delivery of a number of services and functions to all the other components.

Patient information can be clustered into three groups:

- Basic (demographic, personal) data about a patient are necessary for the unique identification within and outside the healthcare organization.
- Patient contacts are events during which the patient has a relationship with the healthcare organization to obtain healthcare services. A contact may be subtyped into ambulatory visits (i.e., outpatient visits), inpatient stays, day clinic, phone consultations, or e-mail exchange.
- Health-related data.

This chapter is only concerned with the first two groups of patient information. Health-related data and their management by the health record component are described in Chapter 6.

Conceptual Specifications

Figure 4.1, using the UML notation, provides a simplified conceptual representation of the patient component. Patient contact data include a start and end time, the reason for admission or transfer, and service points involved in patient care. Every contact is characterized by a state, which may be planned, active, or completed. Administrative data, basic clinical and epidemiologic data, summary (discharge) letters, and administrative notes for insurance companies are all related to a contact. Contacts may be aggregated into cases clustered for clinical and/or organizational purposes (e.g., cycles of care).

Physicians relate to a patient in different roles: attending physician, referring physician, supervising physician, general practitioner, and so on. These roles contain information on physicians and the corresponding specific relationship that may change over time.

"PATIENT"

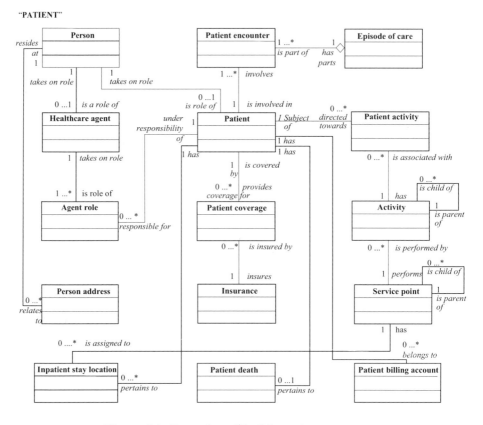

Figure 4.1: General model of the patient component.

Functional Specifications

The patient component provides services to most components of a clinical information system. Almost all services are required to build a patient *admission–discharge–transfer* (ADT) system. The following activities are examples of functions to be supported by the patient component.

Patient Retrieval

Avoiding duplicate registration of patients is a key issue of any clinical information system. Various mechanisms to select a patient should therefore be provided. They include search by patient name, social security number, birthdate, referring physician, waiting lists, and phonetic algorithms (Figure 4.2).

Identification of a patient already in a institution can be done by attending lists, ward units, work lists, and so on.

Event type: patient retrieval
Patient query by name, birthdate, patient unique identifier
Patient query by phonetic search (family or marital name)
Patient query by attending list
Patient query by referring physician
Patient query by work list (radiology modality list, lab working list)
Query for census

Figure 4.2: Patient retrieval functions.

Patient Identification and Registration

Patient identification data can be recorded easily and quickly. Screen logic must be designed to reflect the typical sequence of tasks performed. Where appropriate, the user is prompted with context-sensitive default values.

Event type: identification and registration
Assign a patient unique identifier (PUI)
Change a patient unique identifier
Register a patient
Delete a patient
Merge patient information from two patient identification records
Update patient information
Assign a medical record number

Figure 4.3: Patient registration function.

With the development of large community health information networks (CHINs) it becomes crucial to use adequate identifiers for patients (Figure 4.3) [Kohane 1998]. The use of a national registration number as patient identifier can result in setting up huge databases supplied from multiple sources (medical and nonmedical) and of possible attempted invasion of patient privacy. Examples of unique identifiers are the Social Security numbers (SSN) or the national registration numbers used to identify patient records in northern European countries such as Sweden. To safeguard privacy, many institutions prefer to define their own patient unique identifiers.

Szolovits and Kohane believe that cryptography techniques can be applied with success and discussed two alternative approaches [Szolovits 1994]. The first technique is based on the fact that every individual receives a private key K (different from his SSN) and that every institution receives a public key H. Applying a cryptographic function f, the proper ID of the patient is calculated by the formula ID = $f(K,H)$ and is unique, that is to say, no two patients will have the same key at the same institution. A second technique is based on the assumption that all patients' private keys are held in a centrally organized ID-server established by the government or another trusted organization. Only authorized institutions have access to this server. They can obtain a proper patient ID that is unique to the institution. The patients' private key is unknown to both the patient and the institution. Both techniques illustrate how difficult it is to design a coherent security scheme that meets the requirements of everyone involved.

Event type: patient admission
Admit a patient
Cancel admission
Pending admission
Cancel pending admission
Preadmit a patient
Cancel pre-admission
Update patient information
Merge patient information from two records
Event type: patient arrival
Patient arrives
Cancel patient arrival
Event type: patient discharge
Discharge a patient
Cancel discharge
Pending discharge
Cancel pending discharge
Leave of absence—out (leaving)
Return from leave of absence—in (returning)

Figure 4.4: Patient admission functions.

Patient Admission and Discharge

If the patient's condition requires an admission as an inpatient, the user interface prompts for admission details (Figure 4.4). Under specific circumstances the user is prompted for additional information, for instance if the patient is admitted to the emergency department.

On completion of a patient arrival and inpatient stay, the patient can be discharged from the institution simply by selecting the patient identification from a list of patients.

Patient Tracking and Transfer Functions

The patient's location and status should be known while the patient is in the institution (Figure 4.5). The patient's current status and previous admissions and transfers can be viewed at any time.

Event type: patient tracking
Patient arrives
Cancel patient arrival
Swap two patients
Census updates
Event type: patient tracking
Transfer a patient
Cancel transfer
Pending transfer
Cancel pending transfer
Transfer an outpatient to inpatient
Transfer an inpatient to outpatient
Patient leaves

Figure 4.5: Patient tracking and transfer.

Patient Health Data Cards

Rationale for Using Health Data Cards

A health data card contains computer-readable data. It is provided to health-care professionals and/or patients to facilitate the provision of care. A wide variety of card technologies containing information for patient identification, such as the Social Security number are planned or already used in national large-scale implementations in many European countries such as Belgium, Germany, and France. The (smart) card is both the key used to access the existing information system, to provide the necessary user identification and security requirements, and the carrier of personal data [Pernice 1995a, van der Broek 1997].

The European Commission has been active in this field. The EURO-CARDS concerted action was established to investigate the subject of data card applications in the healthcare system and to reach a consensus on the most suitable strategic approach. EUROCARDS recommends the following priority levels for implementation [Pernice 1995b]:

1. *Healthcare professional cards* enhance the security of healthcare information systems used with or without patient cards, especially if clinical information is stored on patient cards.

2. *Patient emergency cards* support the capacity to host the administrative data for national and international administrative purposes (including the E111 formular).

3. *Patient health data cards* contain medical and pharmaceutical information or pointers to it.

Card Technologies

Various types of card technologies can be combined to allow data to be stored in machine-readable format in a magnetic strip, a bar code, an optical memory strip, an electronic serial memory chip, or a computer chip (Figure 4.6).

Media type	Laser card, optical memory card	Smart IC card (micro-processor)	Magnetic strip card	Floppy diskette (3.5")
Characteristics				
Medium	Optical WORM	Integrated circuit	Magnetic	Magnetic
Recording method	Diode laser	Direct electronic	Electro-magnetic	Electro-magnetic
Erasable data	No	Yes	Yes	Yes
Permanent audit trail	Yes	No	No	No
Updatable records	Yes	Yes	No	Yes
Capacity				
Total capacity	4100 Kbytes	8 Kbytes	0.25 Kbytes	1400 Kbytes
Equivalent number of pages or lines	>1200 pages	4 pages	3 lines	700 pages
Affected by				
Temperatures up to 80°C	No	Variable	Yes	Yes
Electrostatic shock	No	Yes	No	No
Magnetic fields	No	No	Yes	Yes
Flexing/bending	No	Yes	No	Yes

Figure 4.6: Main card technologies.

Cards can be embossed, carry graphics, identification photographs, signature panels, holograms, or combinations of these to discourage fraud.

Obstacles to overcome are the absence of standards on the content and technical level (i.e., standard interfaces that would allow cards manufactured by different suppliers to be read or written on by any card read/write device) although work is being carried out by the CEN TC251 standardization committee.

Examples of Health Data Card Applications

Here are examples of roles played by patient data cards [Maloney 2000]:

- Identification of the patient. The card provides patient identification information that allows the correct match between patient and patient-related data [Panacea 1994].
- Information transfer to synchronize data between incompatible and dispersed information databases.
- Access control to (local or remote) information systems or another card based on the possession of cryptographic class keys indicating the holder professional status.
- Keys for electronic signatures to authenticate the sender. Electronic keys carried on smart cards are considered more secure than keys carried on other media, such as floppy disks.
- Encryption/decryption functions.

Some examples of card programs in the United States and Europe are briefly discussed below.

United States Projects

In 1997 medical division of the Department of Veterans Affairs (VA) implemented a nationwide upgrade of its patient card to an electronically readable card (magnetic strip, bar code, and black and white picture) produced in about one minute, in order to speed patient medical record look-up. These cards function as identifier and data carrier (for a small amount of information), and are personalized at each facility with information downloaded from the hospital information system.

The VA has also developed a demonstration implementation of the G-8 *healthcare data card* interoperability specification. The objective is to demonstrate interoperability with other implementations of this specification such as the Netlink project sites in France, Italy, and Quebec. The VA will also investigate the feasibility of using the PKI (Public Key Infrastructure) keys stored on the G-8 card to interact with Web applications such as electronic application forms and to provide access to copies of the patient's health record.

European Projects

Europe has seen many card programs. Of particular interest are projects carried out in France (Vitale card), Belgium (SIS card), and Germany (Krankenkassekarte). Smart cards have been issued to every citizen registered in the national health scheme [Baylis 2001] .

The French government has completed an ambitious plan: the family insurance card, Carte Vitale. A total of 42 million smart cards were distributed to all insurance policy holders and a large number of healthcare providers in May 1999. In the future, all healthcare providers will be included. In addition, a French healthcare network was launched in November 1998 to facilitate communications between healthcare providers and insurances companies. The French are also piloting an individual card with plans to distribute it to each citizen. This card, Carte Vitale 2, will contain medical data in addition to the identification and insurance data found on Carte Vitale 1. Current plans are to begin distribution in 2003. The French government also initiated the distribution of the healthcare professional card (or CPS) to all 300,000 French healthcare professionals. This card contains a cryptographic chip and securely stores private keys. It will be used to control access to the French healthcare network, to digitally sign documents, and to control access to data contained on patient cards.

The Belgian government has distributed over 10 million cards (SIS cards) to all citizens in 1999 and 2000. These cards function as an identifier and data carrier. The Belgian cards are memory chip cards used primarily for personal and insurance identification. Cards contain a public part and an private part, which can only be read using a digital key. The Belgian Healthcare Network (CareNet) was also launched in 2001 to facilitate communications between hospitals and insurance companies.

Germany has distributed 80 million cards to all citizens in 1994 and 1995. These cards also function as an identifier and data carrier, and are serial memory chip cards used primarily for insurance identification. A reader/printer system allows patient data contained on the card to be automatically printed as a completed insurance form or transferred to a personal computer. There are options to generate and send an electronic submission directly to the insurance fund, eliminating the paper portion of the transaction.

CARDLINK a multi-country, portable medical record project with smart cards (supported by the European Commission-5 with pilot sites in Saint-Nazaire, France; Dublin, Ireland; Milan, Italy; Rome, Italy; and Valencia, Spain), recently concluded its 5-year pilot phase. This card functions as an identifier and data carrier. The data includes emergency data, medications, and pointers to locations where additional patient medical data can be obtained. Approximately 100,000 cards were issued.

Other important projects are EUROCARDS—the European Union (EU) Advanced Informatics in Medicine (AIM) Concerted Action on Data Card Applications in the Healthcare system [Pernice 1995b], and the Trust Health Initiative. The latter is a framework to demonstrate telematic systems using modern security techniques in an open systems connectivity environment with trans-European interoperability. The framework uses smart cards and the RSA asymmetric encryption method to enhance health care information security. The European Commission sponsored and started the project in 1995, which involved nine countries and multiple suppliers.

The G-8 Health Care Data Card Project is one of six healthcare international cooperative initiatives to demonstrate the positive potential of the global information society. This project focuses on an international emergency card, an international harmonized administrative data set, and an international professional card that will allow the secure identification of healthcare professionals when accessing medical data and network services.

Summary and Conclusions

The patient business component is the cornerstone of each medical system and is responsible for the correct identification of the patient, the processing of basic patient data, and the delivery of a number of services to other components. Patient information represents the central issue in the entire healthcare information system, relevant for almost every functional area in supporting the clinical, administrative, and epidemiologic activities.

The basic services provided by the patient business component are

- patient identification and registration;
- maintenance of patient identifiers and related demographic data;
- admission, discharge and transfer;
- bed management scheduling, preadmissions;
- acquisition, storage, and dispatching of referral letters, insurance notifications, certificates, etc.; and
- generation of statistical overviews.

The impact of mobility and connectivity driven by the Internet continues to be felt by organizations throughout the world. Cards are a tool that simplify daily interactions and provide this instant access. However, as confidential information may be stored on the card, privacy and security issues must be considered. This is possible through authentication and encryption techniques. In the healthcare domain, many types of card technologies are already being used for identification or data transfer purposes. The storage of an electronic signature on a smart card provides a means for holder authentication and allows secure access to sensitive information. It is very useful to have essential data, such as electronic keys, identification, and emergency data, stored on the card.

References

[Baylis 2001] Baylis N. E-signatures in healthcare. *e-doc.* 2001; 1(6): 17.

[CEN 1997] CEN/TC251. *PrENV 12967-1. Healthcare Information System Architecture Part 1 (HISA) - Healthcare Middleware Layer.* March 1997. [http://www.centx251.org].

[Kohane 1998] Kohane IS, Dong H, Szolovits P. Health information identification and de-identification toolkit. *Proc AMIA Symp.* 1998; 356–360.

[Maloney 2000] Maloney D. *Health Smart Cards – Looking Back and Looking Forward.* CardTech SecurTech 2000 Conference, May 1–4, 2000; Miami Beach, Florida. [http://www.va.gov/card/presentations.htm].

[Panacea 1994] *Project PANACEA. Overview Version 1.0.* Eureka Funded Programme Consortium, August 1994. [http://www.haldon-house.co.uk/panacea.html].

[Pernice 1995a] Pernice A, Doaré H. International harmonisation of use of data cards in healthcare. *Smart Card Europe Conference,* December 13, 1995. [http://www.va.gov/card/presentations.htm].

[Pernice 1995b] Pernice A, Doaré H, Rienhoff O. Healthcare Card Systems. EUROCARDS Concerted Action Results and Recommendations. *Studies in Health Technology and Informatics.* Amsterdam: IOS Press, 1995; 22: 224.

[Szolovits 1994] Szolovits P, Kohane I. Against simple universal health-care identifiers. *J Am Med Inform Assoc.* 1994; 1(4): 316–319.

[van den Broek 1997] Van den Broek L, Sikkel AJ (eds). Health Cards '97. *Studies in Health Technology and Informatics.* Amsterdam: IOS Press, 1997.

5

The Activity Component

The purposes of patient record keeping are to capture and to communicate the important features of a patient's illness together with the flow of events that occur during health care. Hospitals must therefore rethink and broaden their views of clinical information systems:

- The focus on *patient-centered care* forces institutions to present a single and near real-time view of the patient's relationship to the healthcare system as a whole, bearing in mind that many healthcare functions and information are geographically scattered around the institution.
- The nature of applications becomes *event-based.* An event is a transition state (activity) triggered by an agent. Activities performed or scheduled in one domain—such as a medication prescription—can trigger a number of other applications or users in other domains to perform a related function (alert reminder, etc.).

The *activity component* covers all types of activities that can be performed in a healthcare center. Activities can either relate to a patient (medical action as an instance of the provision of care, directly or indirectly) in the context of a care plan, or relate to the overall organization and administration (nonmedical action) of the healthcare center.

A clinical activity demands tight cooperation and coordination between various users (clinicians, nurses, etc.) and services (specialties) to enhance organizational integration. Therefore, the activity component coordinates business processes (scheduling, conflict prevention, etc.) and interactions among healthcare agents (individual functional units, staff members, software components) related to the requisition, acceptance, planning, and reporting of services. It comprises two important issues: the status of an activity (also known as the activity life cycle), and the corresponding requester-performer relationship between the healthcare agent requesting the activity and the agent performing it.

Conceptual Specifications

Activities and Tasks

In the CEN HISA (Health Information System Architecture) model, an activity is defined as "something which is consciously done, in order to achieve particular results" [CEN 1997]. An activity is generally a provision of healthcare for the benefit of a patient.

An activity requires a set of resources such as medical equipment, personnel, room and time. Activities may use consumable products such as drugs, needles, tubes, photographs, and so on. Activities can be categorized as elementary or composite (protocols) that cluster a number of elementary activities responding to a specific medical need and linked to each other by temporal (performed at different points in time) and other constraints. Examples are radiotherapy treatments of specific tumors necessitating a number of irradiation sessions and CT scans for intermediate evaluation. Some composite activities are repetitive in nature. A drug treatment regimen is an example of a repetitive activity.

Diagnostic activities
Laboratory
Consult
Functional activities (ECG, EEG, ...), ...
Therapeutic activities
Medication
Surgical interventions
Laboratory tests
Preventive procedures, ...
Nursing activities
Vital signs
Wounds
Feeding, ...
Administrative activities
Admission, discharge, transfer
Notification, ...
Logistic activities
Supplier order
Equipment repair order, ...

Figure 5.1: Types of activities.

Activities are carried out at specific service points (departments) that can be considered a cluster of individual resources (time, staff members, equipment, and location). They are set up together to perform a number of classes of activities. Clinical activities related to a patient are an example of the provision of care. They can be classified into three groups (Figure 5.2):

- *Observational activities* generate information on the healthcare status of the patient. This information can be a quantitative result, a descriptive result, or the combination of both.
- *Interventional activities* attempt to change or maintain the health status of the patient.
- *Logistical activities* support the healthcare process, such as admission to a ward unit, meals.

The execution of an activity is governed by the knowledge component (see Chapter 7 for more detail) defining for each activity a number of medical and organizational constraints (rules) and describing the function of an activity throughout its life cycle. Types of links include

- hierarchical links between classes of activities;
- composition links including time constraints;
- interaction links including other constraints, such as interdiction of the execution of other activities within a certain time frame, the preliminary and/or subsequent execution of a set of complementary activities;
- links with quantified resources;
- links with consumable resources; and
- links with temporally constrained resources including points of service and point of service sessions.

Classification of Healthcare Tasks

In general, three broad classes of tasks can be discerned in the medical field:

- *Registering (recording)-oriented tasks* refers to the process of observing and controlling the course of a patient's condition.
- *Reasoning-oriented tasks* concern the search for the hypothesis or explanation (prediction, diagnosis) regarding the patient's condition. In this phase we deal with the semantics of data.
- *Planning-oriented tasks* concern the selection of a set of actions leading to a desired future state (i.e., improved condition of a patient) or leading to additional information on the patient's state in terms of vital signs, and multimedia patient data.

After the previous steps, physicians aim to increase certainty of the derived diagnosis or want to change the health status of the patient. This results in a plan of action: diagnostic procedures in the first case or therapeutic interventions in the second case or even both. If a diagnosis cannot be reached with certainty, a plan of action is established to obtain additional

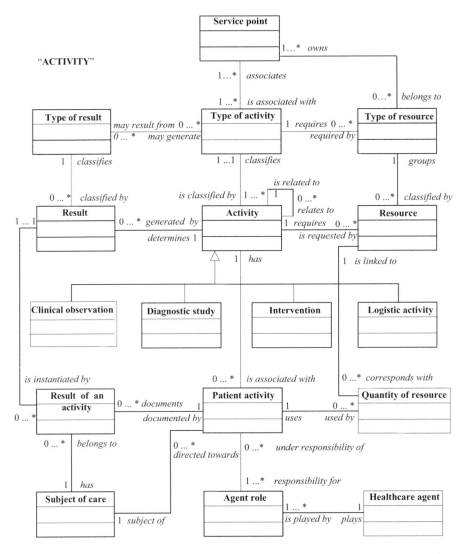

Figure 5.2: Generic activity component.

data. Just as in the reasoning phase, planning can be associated with a number of goals. For instance, a typical goal for therapy planning is the selection of the best therapy for a particular patient, given a number of possible treatments. Other frequent goals in therapy planning are the establishment of the utility of a particular treatment for a particular patient and the selection of prophylactic treatment.

By analogy with linguistic definitions, recording tasks can be associated with the syntactical dimension of tasks, reasoning with the semantic and action definitions, and planning with the pragmatic dimension (Figure 5.3).

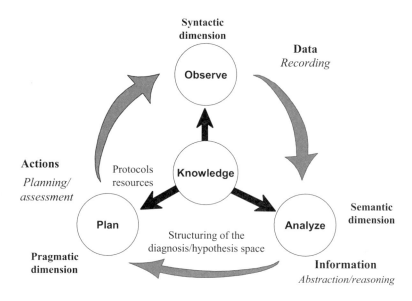

Figure 5.3: The three dimensions of medical tasks.

The Life Cycle of an Activity

An activity can be followed through its life cycle. It changes its status according to different events that may occur: a request, acceptance of a request, rejection, cancellation. Other statuses are holding or delaying, scheduling, performing, validating, and reporting [RICHE 1992]. Activities are initiated by agents (human, software artifact). They might trigger other activities. In the "requester–performer scenario" the initiating agent, generally a healthcare professional (the requester) requests that another professional (the performer) carry out a service for a given patient (Figure 5.4).

A different agent may trigger each state transition. The typical life cycle of an activity may be summarized as follows (Figure 5.5):

- An agent can decide to request a set of activities from other agents of the healthcare organization (e.g., the case of an appointment unit for outpatients accepting requests made by external centers and general practitioners). The requesting agent may or may not belong to the same healthcare organization in which the requested activities will be executed.

- For each group of homogeneous activities, the person making the request (requester) to the service point, which is supposed to deliver the service(s), sends a formal requisition. The requisition details the list of the services that are requested, specifies the reason for the requested service(s), and includes other possible administrative and clinical information, depending on the organization and on the type of requested activities.

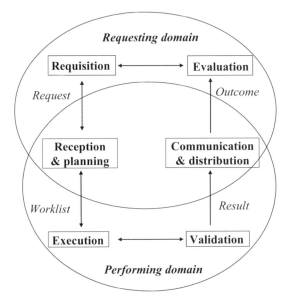

Figure 5.4: Generic workflow structure in a requester/performer scenario.

- When the service provider receives the request, an acknowledgment is sent to the requester, informing the latter of the acceptance of the request and providing or requesting, necessary, other information such as scheduling data.

- Elementary activities are scheduled with the expected date and time of execution. The execution planning is communicated to the requester.

- Even if the delivering service point already schedules activities, some modifications may be performed either by the requester or by the service point, such as the date and time of the activity. Such modifications are usually negotiated between those involved, on the basis of their mutual requirements.

- The service point performs the activity as closely as possible to the scheduled time and date.

- Sometimes some of the requested activities cannot be performed by the service provider, who might decide to forward the request to a different unit, informing the requester of the situation. Such a process may be repeated several times, especially if very complex activities are involved.

- The execution of an activity may last a certain period of time (even several days). A typical case is the service requested by the ADT department to a ward unit for a patient throughout a stay. During this period, intermediate communications may occur between the provider and the original requester.

- The provider, eventually on his/her own initiative, may perform additional activities. Such activities always refer to the original request.

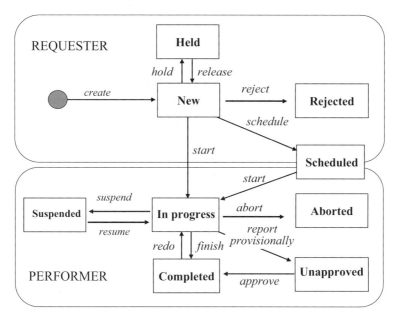

Figure 5.5: Status of an activity in the requester and performer roles. An agent triggers the activity status.

- When the providing unit has completed all activities related to the delivery of the requested service, a final report with the consolidated results of the activity is finalized and the necessary financial elements are generated. The initial request can be considered completed and a formal communication is sent to the requester, who formally acknowledges its receipt.
- Upon execution of an activity, various types of health data may be generated (coded, structured, text, images, etc.). Depending on the type of activity, health data may represent part of the electronic health record or just data to be communicated in the healthcare organization.
- When executing an activity, a set of resources is used such as equipment, staff time, materials, consumables, and so on. The structure of a generic healthcare center is described as a set of service points, being organizational elements (i.e., individuals or complete units), that represent functional aggregations, each of them capable of performing certain activities.

Both the workflow associated with the execution of an activity and the generated information, the result of the act, can be considered as part of the electronic health record.

Provider Order Entry Systems

Computer-based provider order entry (POE)[1] systems are becoming critical in healthcare institutions since they hold potential benefits in terms of improving the quality of patient care and reducing costs [Sittig 1994]. Studies have shown that POE system lead to better accuracy and completeness of medical orders, which in turn lead to reduced lengths of patient stay and costs [Tierney 1993]. They allow fast transmission of orders, legibility, and on-line tracking of the life cycle of an order.

Despite potential benefits, many implementations have not been successful or have failed. Several reasons have been proposed. POE systems are slower to generate orders compared to paper and pen. There are too many screens to create an order, user friendliness is insufficient, and physicians are reluctant to accept POE systems. When launching an order the requester's main concern is time, conflicting sometimes with the interest of the recipient whose highest priority is quality control (on the medical and organizational levels). Speed of input is therefore critical and can be improved in various ways. For example, selecting an item to be ordered could be simplified by entering the first few letters of the item, which would call up a possible list of items for selection.

Benefits

The benefits of POE systems can be categorized as follows:
- Improvement of the healthcare delivery process [Gardner 1990, Hodge 1990, Ogura 1988]
  - Establish the basis for a patient care plan system
  - Eliminate lost orders
  - Eliminate ambiguities caused by illegibility of handwritten orders
  - Generate related orders automatically
  - Track orders and provide feedback about activities provided to the patient as part of the patient's EMR
  - Integrate quality-assurance monitors into the order-capture process
  - Reduce the amount of preprinted forms used in the order entry processes
- Enhanced communication within the institution
  - Faster order handling reduces the time required to initiate and execute orders and phone calls (no need to carry orders around)

[1.] Generally found in the literature under the term *physician order entry* with a "too" narrower meaning.

- Helps organize nurses' work (e.g., the nursing system interacts with the order entry system to help provide a continuum of care [O'Connell 1996])

- Interface with billing systems and materials management

- Co-signing and verifying orders

• Tracing orders through different view mechanisms

- By status: requested, rejected, received, scheduled, in process, performed, reported, or abandoned

- By requesting or performing services (by date)

- By type or by worklist

• Increased cost-consciousness: over 70% of the cost of healthcare is determined by what physicians order in the course of providing patient care; clearly, the most effective way to manage healthcare costs is to provide information and educate physicians regarding cost-effective (medication) options [Kawahara 1989]

- By providing detailed information on order costs when physicians are making decisions through the real-time display of charge/cost data, or by proposing less expensive alternatives [Tierney 1990]

- By helping prescription practices remain consistent with a hospital's policy [Schroeder 1986].

Requirements

Most medical information systems today succeed in making information retrieval more efficient. They frequently fail in terms of physician participation in the direct entry of orders. The requirements that have been found useful in the successful implementation of order entry systems are briefly summarized below.

User Interface Strategies

Coherent if not uniform order entry processes facilitate acceptance by healthcare professionals. This concerns each type of order: medical orders (laboratory, radiology, surgical interventions, etc.), medications and intravenous orders, logistical orders (disposables, meals, etc.), supplier orders, and nursing services.

Menus and screens should be customizable. Users (requesters) should be able to configure their most frequently ordered items in a hierarchical, personal list or "favorites" menu. They should be able to keep their customized context from one session to the next.

It should be possible to enter different types of orders concurrently on one screen via a drag and drop in a workspace area or by double clicking. Highlighting the desired items in a list automatically copies the selected items in the workspace that replicates a paper (unformatted) order document. Default values (e.g., dosage and frequency for medication, etc.) should be easily accessed within each field and be overridden by the user on the fly. Mandatory fields should appear in a different color.

Additional screens can be configured to request additional information according to the item selected.

Once a selection is made, the system can check potential allergies and/or interactions with other drugs currently prescribed for the patient, duplicate tests, and so on.

Information Capture

Two types of entry modes are convenient. Fast order entry modes generate an order with minimum data entry (using text parser, shortcuts), while an extended POE input mode allows a (novice) user to simply enter orders. As order items are selected, the corresponding order-item screen (detail screen) is reconfigured to accommodate the specific ordering attributes of each item. Comments can be attached to orders and links to the patient problem list (multiple problem linkage) can be made.

Spreadsheet Facilities

Physicians and nurses should also be able to group patients according to various selection criteria: worklist, appointment list, personal patients, and so on. This spreadsheet can be used afterward as a starting point to launch a number of orders for that group of patients.

Problem Linkage

Orders for patients can be linked to a specific problem, either automatically by means of data buried in the electronic patient record system, or manually, or a combination of both.

Order Entry Modes

Various order entry modes—dependent on the context of clinical work—are convenient to shorten the time necessary to generate orders:

- Free or unformatted orders can be used for free text recommendations.
- Order sets offer a variety of orders defined by a group of physicians, based on a recommended care plan in the event of the occurrence of a specific pathology, diagnosis, or medical situation in order to achieve an optimized care plan. Plans generate subsequent orders (order sets). Order sets can significantly shorten the time needed to enter orders. Order sets may be activated and then edited. The physician reviews and edits the "order set" to make it appropriate for his patient:

12 lead ECG

CPK, CPK-MB q8h × 3

LDH, LDH-isozyme q12h × 6

- Items (activities, consumables) can be selected by name, or from a catalog using single or multilayered pick lists or menus.
- Templates or fill in the blanks. Templates provide the user with additional capabilities to modify an order or adapt a corresponding order to the specific situation. For example, an admission template could be defined, related to a specific department (ward or unit) or pathology to be treated or any specific situation, generating requests for X-rays, laboratory tests, medication, diagnostic procedures, and so on.
- Completed orders to allow the retroactive entry of orders that have been completed and should not be repeated.
- Change orders (ability to pull up an old order and modify it). Healthcare professionals should be able to reorder (renew automatically with validation), modify, cancel, hold, or discontinue an existing order.

Future-dated orders can be launched effectively and triggered to the destination departments at the appropriate time.

Entry Accesses and Electronic Signatures

To ensure a certain form of security, it must be possible to specify who is allowed to enter the different types of orders: written orders may be entered by licensed MDs, while provisional orders may be entered by medical students. Afterwards these provisional orders must be signed for approval by a licensed MD. The order should be signed electronically by the person responsible for creating it.

The acceptance of verbal orders warrants specific attention and discussion. There is a risk that they could lead to transcription errors, raises the issue of liability and responsibility. They should at least be presented to a professional with sufficient seniority at the next logon.

All modifications should be traceable (e.g., through nondeletion storage techniques). It must be possible to launch orders anywhere, anytime (24 hours a day) if the user has the necessary authorization.

Order Attributes

The main attributes of an order are summarized in Figure 5.6. The link attribute is important to associate orders with problems and prepare evaluation studies.

POE and Computer-Based Decision Support

Since much of a patient's care plan is expressed through orders, the application of clinical decision support in a POE system is a compelling reason for its use by physicians and other health professionals to help prevent certain medical errors and improve accuracy and legibility. Professionals often operate independently, performing a task in isolation without the benefit of knowledge from other team members. A clinical decision support system integrated in an POE system would avoid this isolation.

In 2000, the Institute of Medicine (IOM) issued a report on errors in health care originating with inpatient care, entitled *"To Err Is Human: Building a Safer Health System"* [Kohn 2000]. This report was based on two studies conducted in the 1990s [Bates 1994, Leape1991, Thomas 1999]. The IOM estimates that adverse events occur in 2.9% to 3.7% of hospitalizations, that 8.8% to 13.6% of the adverse events result in patient death, and that more than half of the events are preventable.

Heading	Qualifiers
Patient	*Identifier, name, gender, birthdate, location*
Provider	*Identifier, name, department*
Requester	*Identifier, name, department*
Problem links	*Name, identifier*: required as an indication for any order; should be able to drag a problem from the problem list into the order dialog (ICD-9 codification); linkage to other orders or diagnoses
Order {item}	*Item*: identifier, description *Time*: of order placement *Start date*: absolute or relative, e.g., now (default) in 3 weeks or 2 days after another event *End date*: open-ended orders have no stop date at the prescription time *Frequency*: for activities that are rendered more than once; these orders should be delivered to the provider at an appropriate time before the order is to be carried out; it includes unscheduled orders and recommendations *Urgency/priority indicator*
Additional information	For example pregnancy, fitted with a pacemaker

Figure 5.6: Attributes of a medical order.

Failure to diagnose was cited as the most frequent error in health care. Medication errors represent the second most common and second most expensive error in health care. The initiation of logic can be active or passive. Active logic is initiated by different kinds of trigger events, a timed event, or a database filing event. A passive event is user-initiated. Three kinds of medical decision support systems (DSSs) are generally considered: critiquing systems, consulting systems, and reminder systems.

Critiquing Systems

Critiquing systems address specific therapeutic or diagnostic activities. Control of the appropriateness of an order, reflecting the various impacts an order may have on other domains such as financial, quality of care, and resource utilization, is an example. For instance, when an activity is requested the DSS may be used to verify its suitability for the patient:

- Is this activity compatible with patient's sex, age, condition?
- Is the patient available at the time requested for this activity?
- Are the hospital resources (staff, equipment) available to perform the activity at the requested time?
- Is this drug contraindicated?

Consulting Systems

Consulting systems assist the clinician in making optimized choices or provide access to disease-based information. Examples are the automatic suggestions of therapeutic or diagnostic orders as part of a medical protocol or automatic suggestions of a dose or alternative drug based on patient weight or body surface area. Another example is assistance in performing complex calculations (drug dosage or parenteral and enteral feeding based on age, weight, and sex).

Reminder Systems

Reminder systems give feedback and highlight preventive actions. The basic methods associated with the DSS mentioned above are the following:

- Substitute checks: recommend alternatives.
- Parameter checks: verify the components of orders such as dose or the frequency.
- Utilization checks: ensure that some tests (laboratory, radiology etc.) are not ordered too frequently in a certain time period or that the accumulated doses of a specific drug do not surpass a certain dosage limit.
- Relevant information displays: present valuable patient information such as lab results (high-low flags for laboratory results) or allergies when specific orders are created.
- Time-based reminders are event-triggered. If the time period expires before another event is generated, the appropriate user is notified. Examples are expired (medication) orders that are not reviewed, or drug levels that have not been checked within a reasonable length of time.

Examples of order-related checking methods are given in Figure 5.7 [Evans 1990, Metzger 2001, Ogura 1988].

Order entry features	Link with the patient record	Link with reference tables
Drug adjustment (check dose against)		
Age, bodyweight, body surface area	+	
Laboratory results	+	
Diagnosis	+	
Cumulative dose limits	+	+
Min.-max. dose ranges		+
Interaction checking		
Drug-drug		+
Drug-allergy	+	+
Drug-disease	+	+
Drug-food	+	+
Advanced checking ordering features		
Automatic start/stop orders (e.g., prophylactic antibiotics)		+
Order sets management (e.g., chemotherapy, parenteral nutrition, disease oriented protocols)	+	+
Suggest associate orders (corollary orders)		+
Impact on cost and quality		
Search for alternative orders (e.g., generic drugs)		+
Search for duplicate orders within a specified time frame	+	
Focus attention on expiring orders	+	
Link to appropriate clinical guidelines		+
Search/request for clinical justification	+	
Order validation (e.g., pharmacy)	+	
Display relevant order information (e.g., dosage, administration, precautions)		+
Display relevant patient data	+	

Figure 5.7: General overview of order entry and checking features.

Event Engine

This paragraph describes, as an example of the functions of an event engine, the architecture of the decision system that has been included in the POE systems of the AZ-VUB University Hospital in Brussels (see Chapter 11). It was inspired by the work of the Brigham and Women's Hospital, Boston, MA (USA) [Hiltz 1994, Teich 1998, 1999b].

When an event occurs (ordering medication, filing a lab result, automatic passing of a deadline, etc.), a *trigger program* is expected to create a message composed of clinical data and trigger parameters that are forwarded to a clinical event monitor. The clinical event monitor logs the trigger messages with appropriate contextual information. An alarm may be generated by the clinical event monitor (e.g., abnormal lab results) or by another application (co-sign orders, approve letter for a general practitioner).

One or more trigger classes (and subclasses) describe the trigger event and are included in the parameter section of the message. Trigger classes group conditions based on the type of data the condition evaluates. The trigger event is responsible for the initiation of the event engine process in the *inference engine*. Trigger classes may be subdivided into multiple subclasses (Figure 5.8).

Allergy orders Create	Lab result Create
Consult order Create	Medication order Create order End order Get name
Deferred event Now	Micro result Create
Diagnosis Create	Registration
Lab order Create	Transfer order Create

Figure 5.8: Trigger classes (e.g., medication order, lab results) are subdivided into multiple subclasses (e.g., filer, get name).

The mechanism of inheritance is applied to rules and several rules may apply to a trigger instance. For example, a penicillin-order trigger may inherit the inference rules associated with both medications and allergens.

The clinical event monitor sends these messages to the inference engine. The inference engine acts on each message individually. Processing can happen synchronously or in the background (asynchronously) to do the following:

1. Analyze the trigger message passed by the clinical event monitor.
2. Determine if the trigger instance meets the conditions for an alert.
3. Invoke a rule within the inference engine.

If the inference engine undertakes any action, it returns the result (alert) to the *notification engine*, which initiates the appropriate response of alerts generated by the inference engine. Reminders for non life-threatening events must not interrupt the clinician.

The alert is displayed in textual form. The concurrency of an alert defines the way it is visualized: synchronous mode or background, asynchronous mode. Asynchronous alerts occur when a user is not available and the trigger is usually a database filing procedure such as an abnormal laboratory result (Figure 5.9).

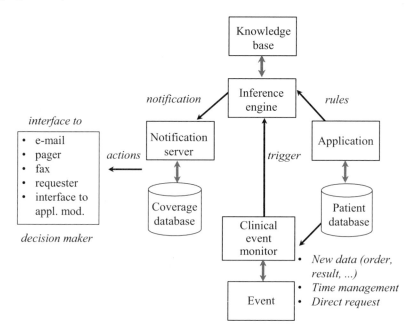

Figure 5.9: Architecture of an order entry decision support system.

No direct action is needed and the processing speed is not an issue. Communication is achieved via e-mail or a pager.

Synchronous alerts are generated when an action from a user connected to a workstation is needed (e.g., drug–lab interaction, drug–drug, cost-based reminder). The notification server logs information about the alert but also the user's response (cancellation of an order). The recipient of an asynchronous alert acknowledges it by reading the certified e-mail and may perform several actions (Figure 5.10). In the notification phase an escalation procedure has to be implemented.

Postpone the action to be undertaken.
Not my patient. Reassigns responsibility for the patient to the correct doctor. The program repeats the alert to another physician.
Act now. Depending on the rule, the recipient may invoke preset actions like ordering specific lab tests or changing medication orders, may call the order entry program for any of its functions, or may simply say "OK, I'll take care of it." The most demanding actions are order, sign, and reply.

Figure 5.10: Acknowledgment of an alert.

Rules

Rules remain the easiest and most common method of description of actions. Main attributes are depicted in Figure 5.11..

Title: the title of the rule.
Enable: determines when the rule runs. It may be active or inactive (on or off). If active, it may run on randomly selected patients or on randomly selected health-care professionals (physicians, nurses) involved with a trigger event (e.g., the healthcare professional who writes an order for a lab test). The notifier may be enabled or disabled separately. While testing a rule, the rule is enabled but the notifier is disabled to permit the designer to examine the results of executing the rule without alerting the caregivers.
Logic: names the conditions that constitute the rule, sets their properties, and groups them into lists that determine the Boolean logic of the rule.
Message: a line of text describing the problem detected by the rule to the person who reads the notifier's announcement. For example, "Patient on Coumadin and anabolic steroids—possible elevated PT."
Notification: how and when the notifier should deliver its announcement. The medium may be certified e-mail, a note on the clinical monitor, a pager, or combinations of these invoked at given times after the rule was fired. Different announcements may pertain to repeated alerts on the same patient when the condition is getting worse or when it is resolving.
Actions: specific actions for the notifier to offer the person receiving the alert, for example, to order a particular lab test or to discontinue a medication.
Triggers: what trigger instances will invoke the rule, and how the rule will run. For example, "run the rule synchronously when someone orders Coumadin" or "run the rule asynchronously when the lab files a prothrombin result."
Report classes: place the rule in one or more report classes, which do not affect the execution of the rule but do group similar rules for reporting. The names and composition of the report classes are the designer's choices.
Delayed effects: name another rule to run later. For example, an order for TPN triggers a rule that causes another rule to check at 10:00 a.m. the next morning whether the TPN order has been renewed. Delayed effects were once called side effects, a term that remains in the names of some subroutines and variables.
Owner and editors: the creator of a rule is its owner. The owner may edit the rule and delegate editing authority to one or more others.
Versioning: each rule is identified by a version ID. Only the latest version is active.

Figure 5.11: Rules attributes.

Production rules indicate that if conditions or premises are met, the conclusions may be affirmed. The conclusions may be a diagnostic hypothesis or an action (additional exams, indication of a treatment, etc.).

IF<conditions>THEN<conclusion>

For example, a rule consists of one list and the list contains two conditions: "patient on potassium acetate" and "patient had BUN ordered in last *n* days." Each condition would have its own set of trigger events, such as the ordering of a medication and the filing of a lab order. The user may decide that the rule should be performed only when ordering a medication so only that trigger event would be selected. A rule must have at least one trigger event selected if it is to be invoked.

Conditions ← *consists of* Rule ←*triggers* Class

Trigger Class ← *consist of* Trigger Events

The other part of the rule definition states what is to happen if the rule is true. This includes notification and action choices. The notify option specifies who and how people are notified, for example by pager, certified e-mail, or simply logging the information. Levels of urgency can be defined, for example, initial, repeat (worse), and repeat (resolving), allowing escalation.

The action function allows a professional to see and respond to all outstanding alerts. It describes the alert and provides a list of actions that can be performed. Examples of possible actions are check a medication order or place a specific order set

Computer-Based Guidelines

The goal in medicine is to reduce the barriers separating research and published literature from clinical practice [Coiera 1997]. Protocols attempt to bridge this gap and to convert this know-how *formally* into clinical practice leading to *evidence-based medicine* (EBM). In this way, others who may have less experience can follow these protocols and ensure that the same high standards are applied in a consistent fashion. Protocols hold together all the elements of care and treatment that each staff member involved needs to deliver within a specified time frame, ensuring that a patient is getting a minimum standard of care at all times and that no patients fall through the net [NTIA 2000].

A protocol can be designed within a specific medical context for a specific diagnosis or case group. A protocol is used in a three-loop model:

1. *Protocol selection* based on a number of entry criteria: contextual variables such as the medical state of the patient, treatment goals, availability of resources needed in terms of consumable, tangible, and intangible resource.
2. *Performance* of the instructions defined and registration of the measurements and variances in the protocol.
3. *Outcome assessment* over a statistically significant number of patients.

As the patient progresses through the protocol the physician has the option of reviewing the exact path taken through the decision tree. For every patient, relevant data generated are stored as part of the electronic health record (EHR) for medical, audit, clinical, or statistical research purposes, and any change from this protocol is registered as a variation. These variations allow analysis, enabling users to modify protocols so that optimal care is always provided.

Protocol-directed care has several advantages. It assists in research by providing the basis on which to judge the effectiveness of (sometimes inherently complex) protocols, assists in the delegation and demarcation of responsibility, and allows dealing with complex and uncommon medical situations. Moreover, it prohibits the more expensive (or unproven) options for managing patients.

Protocols establish the need for rather complicated computer assistance because they do the following:

- Guide clinicians in making better decisions by selecting the best protocol of treatment for a patient.
- Result in more efficient and automated workflow mechanisms (order entry and activity scheduling).
- Provide healthcare details automatically recorded in the EHR. In every "decision point" of the protocol the system could generate task-specific data entry displays that can influence the next healthcare task to be undertaken.
- Support electronic reminders, alerts, or warnings and may monitor medical devices.

However, the real challenge is found in the architectural implementation on the technical and medical levels. On the technical level, a computer-based protocol cannot be designed as a "rigid" protocol but as a flexible system that can be changed on the fly depending on the changing medical condition of the patient. Several guideline formalisms are available: decision tables, Arden syntax, EON, Prestige (UK), Prodigy (UK), and GLIF. On the medical level, protocols are not a one-time event but an ongoing process necessitating continuing refinement and modification.

Framework for Automating Medical Processes: The Workflow Engine

Continuity of care requires a cooperative environment among autonomous complementary medical departments in terms of data and functions. In the realm of activity management, this component can be associated with the workflow mechanism that plays an important role in automating medical processes. This engine is necessary to trigger the various action rules at the right time in the business process life cycle.

A *workflow engine* facilitates business processes in which information among different partners must be mutually exchanged according to a defined set of business rules in order to achieve or to contribute to an overall business goal [Hollingsworth 1995]. Processes may have life cycles ranging from minutes (results reporting, order requests, appointments, reminders, etc.), to days (certificates), or to months (cervical cancer screening). Processes can also used for pre-fetching images in the domain of radiotherapy and nuclear medicine.

The main elements of the workflow engine are the rules to be followed at the decision points. They are briefly explained in Figure 5.12.

Decision points	Business processes may include multiple processing paths. The system must provide a way to select the appropriate processing path for each transaction.
Business rules	Rules are the hospital's business practices reflected in software, and they define the activities required for each process and for the routing (when, where) of business data.
Roles	A role is a class of user who shares the same type of work.
Routing	Routing connects the activities in the workflow. It is an instruction that tells the system to forward information to the next step in the business process. It specifies what information to forward and where to forward it.
Work lists	Work lists are lists of (ordered) work items awaiting a particular activity as part of a business process. The following issues are addressed: • *Prioritization of work items* For example, in a pharmacy, it is possible to prioritize work items on the basis of the type of medication required or from the oldest to the newest requisition. • *Pooled lists or specific assignments* Worklists are allocated to users assigned to a particular role or are created by assigning specific items to specific users or roles. For example, all CT requests can be grouped into a CT worklist, or results from biopsies or a range of medical results can be sent to a particular physician, so that the physician "owns" the result relationship. • *Timeout exception processing* The system can automatically reassign work items to other worklists if they've been sitting around for too long.
Business events	Business events cause changes to business objects or the state of the business process (transition from one task of a business process to another). They may occur as a result of a change in the value of critical data (e.g., abnormal blood result), a due date that has passed, or a condition that tells the system an activity is complete. Business events create workflow that integrates applications through a technique called *publish and subscribe*. Publishers trigger an event, while subscribers are dependent on the publishing of an event.

Figure 5.12: Elements and requirements of a workflow engine.

Summary and Conclusions

The activity component is the most important cornerstone in achieving integration within the patient's healthcare process. Integration aims to supply organizational integration and not simply connect systems or departments. Hence the activity component must reflect and support the medical organization as a whole.

The activity component enhances organizational integration by coordinating the flow of work (and information) between various healthcare professionals, by enabling coordinated care planning, scheduling (as part of the resource component), and tracing possible conflicts.

Many argue that the greatest long-term benefit of POE systems comes from the integration of clinical decision support systems in the order-entry process [McDonald 1976, Pryor 1990]. Despite considerable benefits, few hospitals have POE systems completely or partially installed because the costs of customizing and implementing "off the shelf" POE packages can be very high. Another obstacle to POE systems is that many physicians resist the idea of ordering prescriptions via computer.

POEs that lack decision support capabilities may have a smaller impact on hospital charges than those that offer decision support [Weiner 1999]. The most economically compelling application of computers to decrease resource utilization in health care is found in the automated generation of alerts, reminders, and suggestions when standards of care (compliance with preventive care protocols) are not being achieved. A recent study in the *Journal of the American Medical Association* estimates that adverse drug reactions are so widespread in the United States that they would fall somewhere between the nation's fourth to sixth leading cause of death. In the medical world where information overload is a real problem, knowledge-based systems will provide savings by highlighting errors, inefficiencies, and wasted money in patient care. "Health care understands that it needs to manage the information process," says Margaret Amatayukul, vice-president of Sheldon Dorenfest & Associates, "but it doesn't value information as an integral part of its core business, unlike banking or airlines which couldn't do without it. In health care, information is used more often to run the business than to deliver the primary product" [Menduno 1998].

POE systems also need to be integrated with a hospital-wide resource scheduling system and the EMR, so that orders may be tracked as part of a patient's health record (see Chapters 6 and 8).

The movement of clinical evidence into clinical practice through the creation of clinical protocols represents a major technical challenge and a promising opportunity in the field of medical informatics. The activity component is an important element of these clinical protocol systems. As is often the case in medical informatics, this type of system will only succeed if it can integrate smoothly with other systems and provide features to register the context within which the protocol will be used.

References

[Amberg 1996] Amberg M, Graber S. Specifying hospital information systems using business process modeling. *Studies in Health Technology and Informatics*, 1996; 34: 1037–1041.

[Bates 1994] Bates DW, O'Neil AC, Boyle D, Teich J, Chertow GM, Komaroff AL, Brennan TA. Potential identifiability and preventability of adverse events using information systems. *J Am Med Inform Assoc.* 1994; 1(5): 404–411.

[CEN 1997] CEN/TC251. *PrENV 12967-1. Healthcare Information System Architecture Part 1 (HISA) - Healthcare Middleware Layer.* Brussels: CEN TC251, March 1997. [http://www.centx251.org].

[Coiera 1997] Coiera E. *Guide to Medical Informatics, the Internet and Telemedicine.* New York: Oxford University Press, 1997.

[Evans 1990] Evans RS, Pestotnik SL, Burke JP, Gardner RM, Larsen RA, Classen DC. Reducing the duration of prophylactic antibiotic use through computer monitoring of surgical patients. *DICP.* 1990; 24(4): 351–354.

[Field 1990] Field M J, Lohr KN (eds). *Clinical Practice Guidelines: Directions for a New Program.* Institute of Medicine (IOM). Washington: National Academy Press, 1990.

[Gardner 1990] Gardner RM, Golubjatnikov OK, Laub RM, Jacobson JT, Evans RS. Computer-critiqued blood ordering using the HELP system. *Comput Biomed Res.* 1990; 23(6): 514–528.

[Hiltz 1994] Hiltz FL, Teich JM. Coverage list: a provider-patient database supporting advanced hospital information services. *Proc Annu Symp Comput Appl Med Care.* 1994; 809–813.

[Hodge 1987] Hodge MH. History of the TDS Medical Information System. *Proc ACM Conf on History of Medical Informatics.* New York: ACM Press, 1987; pp. 143–152.

[Hollingsworth 1995] Hollingsworth D. *Workflow Management Coalition. The Workflow Reference Model.* Document Number TC00-1003. Version 1.1. Winchester, Hampshire, UK: WFMC, 1995. [http://wfmc.org/standards/docs.htm].

[Kawahara 1989] Kawahara NE, Jordan FM. Influencing prescribing behavior by adapting computerized order-entry pathways. *Am J Hosp Pharmacol.* 1989; 46(9): 1798–1801.

[Kohn 2000] Kohn LT, Corrigan JM, Donaldson MS (eds). *To Err is Human: Building a Safer health System.* Institute of Medicine (IOM). Washington: National Academy Press, 2000.

[Leape 1991] Leape LL, Brennan TA, Laird N, Lawthers AG, Localio AR, Barnes BA, Hebert L, Newhouse JP, Weiler PC, Hiatt H. The nature of adverse events in hospitalised patients: results of the Harvard Medical Practice Study II. *N Engl J Med.* 1991; 324(6): 377–384.

[McDonald 1976] McDonald CJ. Protocol-based computer reminders, the quality of care and the non-perfectibility of man. *N Engl J Med.* 1976; 295(24): 1351–1355.

[Menduno 1998] Menduno M. Software that plays hardball—expert clinical systems fend off forgetfulness, mistakes, and fraud investigators. *Hospitals & Health Networks.* 1998; 5: 46–48.

[Metzger 2001] Metzger J, Turisco F. *Computerized Physician Order Entry: A Look at the Vendor Marketplace and Getting Started,* December 2001. Long Beach, CA: First Consulting Group [http://www.fcg.com/webfiles/pdfs/CPOE_Guide.pdf].

[NTIA 2000] NTIA. U.S. Department of Commerce. *Falling through the net. Toward Digital Inclusion,* October 2000. Washington: National Telecommunication and Information Administration – US Department of Commerce [http://search.ntia.doc. Gov.].

[O'Connell 1996] O'Connell EM, Teich JM, Pedraza LA, Thomas D. A comprehensive inpatient discharge system. *Proc AMIA Annu Fall Symp.* 1996; 699–703.

[Ogura 1988] Ogura H, Sagara E, Iwata M. On-line support functions of prescription order system and prescription audit in an integrated hospital information system. *Medical Informatics.* 1988; 13: 161–169.

[Pryor 1990] Pryor AT, Dupont R, Clay J. A MLM based order entry systems. *Proc 14th Annu Symp Comput Appl Med Care.* 1990; 579–583.

[RICHE 1992] RICHE Consortium. *RICHE ESPRIT project.* Final Report. November 30, 1992 [http://www.newcastle.research.ec.org/esp-syn/text/2221.html].

[Schroeder 1986] Schroeder CG, Pierpaoli PG. Direct order entry by physicians in a computerized hospital information system. *Am J Hosp Pharmacol.* 1986; 43(2): 355–359.

[Sittig 1994] Sittig DF, Stead WW. Computer-based physician order entry: the state of the art. *JAMA.* 1994; 1(2): 108–123.

[Teich 1998] Teich JM. Clinical information systems for integrated healthcare networks. *Proc AMIA Symp.* 1998; 19–28.

[Teich 1999a] Teich J. Inpatient order management. *J Healthcare Information Management.* 1999; 13(2): 97–110.

[Teich 1999b] Teich JM, Glaser JP, Beckley RF, Aranow M, Bates DW, Kuperman GJ, Ward ME, Spurr CD. The Brigham integrated computing system (BICS): advanced clinical systems in an academic hospital environment *Int J Med Inf.* 1999; 54(3): 197–208.

[Tierney 1990] Tierney WM, Miller M., McDonald CJ. The effect on test ordering of informing physicians of the charges for outpatient diagnostic tests. *N Engl J Med.* 1990; 322(21): 1499–1504.

[Tierney 1993] Tierney WM, Miller ME, Overhage JM, McDonald CJ. Physician inpatient order writing on microcomputer workstations. Effects on resource utilization. *JAMA.* 1993; 269(3): 379–383.

[Thomas 1999] Thomas EJ, Studdert DM, Newhouse JP, et al. Costs of medical injuries in Utah and Colorado. *Inquiry.* 1999;36: 255–264.

[Weiner 1999] Weiner M, Gress T, Thiemann DR, Jenckes M, Reel SL, Mandell SF, Bass EB. Contrasting views of physicians and nurses about an inpatient computer-based provider order-entry system. *J Am Med Inform Assoc.* 1999; 6(3): 234–244.

6

The Health Record Component

*The passive medical records of today's
information systems must change into
active objects. Medical information processing is not an end in and of itself. It is
essential that we bear in mind that the
patient is the subject of care with a problem, not the health care system.*

—D.J. De Brota, 1994

Scope of Health Records

The *health record component* is dedicated to the acquisition, storage,
retrieval, processing and communication (interchange) of patient-related
health data. The term *health data* is understood in a broad sense since it
includes different kinds of health-related information such as patients' habits,
family history, nursing, biologic data, medical images, genetic information,
and so on. It is directly related to the management of the *electronic health
record* (EHR). Its content includes the medical record, as created and used by
physicians, the nursing record, and the specialized records used by the various health professionals and social workers [Iakovidis 1998]. Until recently
the terms *electronic patient record* (EPR) and *electronic medical record*
(EMR) were the most frequently used terms to express the multiplicity and
diversity of heath-related information.

According to the GEHR (Good European Health Record) project consortium, a health record is "a collection of information and facts set down in
writing, or pictorially or in electronic format as a means of preserving knowledge" [GEHR 1993]. Furthermore, it is a deletionless logbook of statements
and health data about patients registered at a certain point in time by a healthcare professional. It should be accessible at any time and place by authorized
healthcare professionals and should be shared across heterogeneous systems
to meet legal and security requirements. Departmental systems focusing on
the needs of only a specific structure are excluded.

In summary, health records are instantiations of an almost infinite number of health concepts composed of rich multimedia data types and their relations encompassed in a wide lattice of terms.

As a "by-product" of the delivery of health actions, health records are now expected to trace the patient/citizen *over space and time* from cradle to grave, providing health information collected at each location of the patient. The health status of a subject of care is described in terms of symptoms or complaints, medical history, observed signs, ordered and performed tests, and underlying pathophysiological states or syndromes. This health record is the central source of data and medical knowledge in the patient's care process.

The architecture of an electronic health record (EHR) system is based on the following three axes:

1. The scope of the health record system functions. These functions vary from supporting human memory, to assisting in medical decision-making and supporting workflow management.
2. The way health records are structured. The topology of clinical/health information (statements) in the health record can be organized chronologically, in a problem-oriented fashion, and so on.
3. The way data are entered or represented in the health record. The granularity of clinical/health statements varies from text-oriented (unstructured) through section-oriented (semi-structured), to content-oriented (coded) structures.

Strategies in Evolving Toward Electronic Health Records

From Healthcare Provider to Patient-Centered Electronic Records

A long-term goal for healthcare institutions is the achievement of life long, longitudinal electronic health records that include all types (text, wave forms, voice, images, and other pictorial information) and forms (clinical, financial, and administrative) of structured information. EHR systems offer many advantages when compared to manual systems. In 1988 McDonald stated that the complete computerization of a medical record was only a matter of time, and that in the meantime, hybrid computerized and paper records had significant advantages over paper-only systems [McDonald 1988]. However, attitudes about patient record systems differ from one institution to the next and among individuals in the same institution.

There is an important trend today to shift from a "healthcare provider–centered record to a computer-based, virtual, longitudinal patient-centered record [De Moor 1994]. The first EHRs were created as individual records in a single physician–patient or health unit–patient relationship. Difficulties with local systems began to arise only when the systems started to communicate. The elimination of geographic barriers with the development of networks and the Internet, and the increased mobility of patients requires reconsidering the ways EHRs are designed and structured. The integration of heterogeneous medical applications becomes a central issue. Data need to be mapped between different application domains, organized according to the way it is perceived by every medical/health department.

Nowadays most information that is shared in clinical information systems is almost never "re-purposed" [Tuttle 1994], meaning that it is almost never reused for other purposes than that for which it was registered. This demand for reusing and sharing data generated in one application in another one, the advent of decision support systems, and the use of intelligent adaptable user interfaces make it necessary to define terminologic servers to share a common model of understanding of the concepts that will be communicated.

The long-term goal of an EHR system should be seen not only in the improved registration of health data but also in the incremental acquisition (generation and representation) of knowledge associated with and derived from medical data based on a standardization of health-related terms and concepts. The passive nature of today's health record systems will gradually have to change into active objects that generate reminders, suggest alternatives, and so on.

Barriers to the Development of Electronic Health Records

Trials on the automation of hospital information systems have demonstrated how complex and difficult it is to computerize health records. EHR requirements often conflict from one professional to the next.

- Health professionals expect user-friendly, low cost, and adaptable systems.
- Developers demand harmonization of user demands, fair prices for their products, and collaboration in areas where competition is counterproductive.
- Patients demand that their health data be transportable and secure.
- Researchers and governments are interested in the quality of aggregated data for epidemiology and peer review.

The reasons for the few successful implementations of EHRs have been analyzed. They include:

- The *lack of understanding* of the nature of clinical practice by systems developers. This is represented by the fact that although administration and organization structures change over time, the fundamental processes of clinical practice remain basically the same [Rector 1995].

- Overly *high expectations* by users and developers in an attempt to get all the possible benefits obtainable from computerization immediately. What cannot be expressed with a certain level of technology should not be implemented [Kuperman 1990].
- Too much *focus on purely technologic issues* (choice of programming languages, databases, networking, etc.) instead of methodologic, applicative, and organizational issues.
- *Lack of agreement* between health professionals on the structure under which information must be or should be kept and for how long.
- *The lack of involvement of health professionals* when applications are put into practice.

Requirements for the Implementation of EHR Systems

The transition from handwritten paper medical records to electronic health records is intrinsically linked to the following challenging issues:

- The development of a *(standard) healthcare record architecture* within a healthcare organization providing a generalized mechanism for describing the items of an EHR, its data content, and structure. The higher the number of users sharing and using EHRs within an institution, the more it becomes important to share a common structure to integrate, communicate, compare, aggregate, and present information in various formats and to provide the users with an integrated perception of the information useful for their practice.
- *Merging* the EHR component with the other health information system components and in particular the patient, activity, and resource components. Most information contained in the EHR is captured in the context of requesting or performing a health activity. Hence each item of information exists in relation to the state of the originating activity.
- A *common medical terminology*. To avoid incompatibilities and to guarantee the consistency, reusability, and sharability of the different components of a larger system, a common understanding of the underlying concepts that describe the care process must be provided. Such shared concept systems are defined as "ontologies or "terminology servers" [Rector 1995] (see Chapter 7). But the implementers of medical terminologies confront difficult challenges. There is no unified view and the number of terms is huge: more than 100,000 basic concepts in medicine and some million terms, frequently used in combined form or with modifiers. Current classification and coding systems (e.g., ICD-9-CM, SNOMED, READ) are either inappropriate or insufficient to record the detail required for acceptable clinical use. Both this lack of a common terminology and the easy linking to knowledge sources hampers the development of EHRs. This demonstrates the importance of developing controlled vocabularies and terminology services to be coupled with the EHR component.

- The increased availability of *communication facilities* to internal and external healthcare providers (e.g., general practitioners, other healthcare organizations). As our society is becoming increasingly mobile, it is necessary for health data to become portable, and as a result software components need to be mail-enabled. This implies the capability of describing the structure of the data elements to be exchanged.

- An *adequate formalization of medical knowledge* to accommodate users with more intelligent features, such as access to knowledge bases, electronic libraries, and the integration of *decision support systems* in order to be able to generate alerts and reminders for health professionals (synchronously or asynchronously), contrasted with manual records, which potentially pinpoint events *after* they have occurred.

- The availability of an *audit trail* to facilitate the detection of data alteration and to address potential security violations. As health records must incorporate a facility to reconstruct their status at any time, a *deletionless* (only amendments are allowed) storage architecture is a key issue. Features of EHR that safeguard security, confidentiality, reliability, user access (user profiles), and data access must be provided.

- *Scalability.* Multidisciplinary institutions require an EHR system that can readily scale as the institution grows while maintaining local ownership of data.

- The automatic availability of a central comprehensive *information repository* for healthcare policymakers (providers, hospital managers) to define future policies by analyzing the past on several levels. Important parameters such as financial data and resources used are buried in the health record. The ability to aggregate these detailed data elements along various axes provides an adequate basis for

  - quality assurance (quality of care against effective resources used and minimal cost);

  - enhanced efficiency through human and material resource planning;

  - financial planning and more accurate billing procedures;

  - classification and grouping of patients;

  - statistical analyses for retrospective and prospective studies based on health record reviews, within an individual record and across populations; and

  - patient and health professional education.

Conceptual Specifications

EHR systems need features to improve readability and to explore the stored information. Health data in the EHR can be divided into two categories: the time dimension and the specificity of health data (Figure 6.1). The information in a health record is a cumulative care profile, made up of various records created with each patient contact, describing the condition of the contact and the resources used.

Time and Events

The health record can be projected on a time line that provides an overview of events for the patient. The user may want to use this overview to obtain more detailed data.

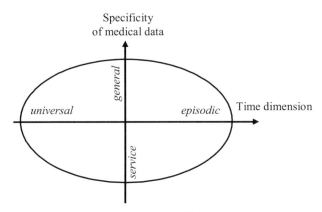

Figure 6.1: Types of clinical data.

Events occur when the healthcare professional interacts with the EHR component. These events

- relate to a single patient;
- are registered at one moment;
- are discovered at one moment; and
- originate with and are under the responsibility, authorization, and authentication of a responsible physician.

Several items of information need to be identified for each event:

- the subject of care,
- the location of the patient (e.g., a medical department, at home),
- the health service provider,
- the time period,
- the specialist service request(s) or requesters,
- the source of the corresponding information,
- the copy destination (zero or more),
- the item version, and
- the access and modification rights.

All clinical data in an EHR should exist only within events. A typical example of an event is a patient contact (or consultation). An event may also reflect interactions with the EHR when the patient is not present in a health unit, such as filing a laboratory result, writing a letter, or obtaining information through a phone call. A simple event (e.g., a patient contact) may lead to one or more health activities (physical exam, history, etc.). An event manager makes use of the structure defined in the system and allows navigation through appropriate screens.

Events also constitute a safe basis for exchanging healthcare record data in shared care environments. An event

- is a unique object of information (it enables safe merging of data from various sources);
- conveys information on the context of the information production (organization and presentation of the data, references to the term sets/models, healthcare enterprise and agent); and
- conveys information facilitating the implementation of ethical-legal regulations (responsibility, authentication, access privileges, management of modified versions).

Events can be subdivided as follows:

- *Management events* [Johnson 1997]

  - *Inpatient management event*: admission, discharge, transfer

  - *Outpatient encounter*: emergency room visit, ambulatory visit

- Clinical events

  - *Contact/encounter* (visit): Information relating to the provision of care by a clinician in contact with a patient, such as physical examination, history, risk factors, medication, and so on. A contact/encounter may apply to several problems while an episode is normally related to one problems. All progress notes can be linked to these encounters and displayed accordingly [Bainbridge 1996].

  - *Results*: Incoming test results, reports, notes made by a clinician about the patient sometimes without patient contact (e.g., laboratory data).

  - *Reminder*: Used by a clinician to record those entries that are important to see on first accessing the patient's record or generated by a decision support system.

  - *Order plan*: All requests launched on behalf of a patient. The content of this event describes future care planned for a certain period.

  - *Letter (episode) summary*: Discharge letter, referral letter, progress notes, relates to past care up to the moment of performance (e.g., coding).

  - *Treatment*: Surgical intervention, drug treatment, radiotherapy, immunization.

  - *Problem*: Definition of a patient's problem.

Events do not contain other events. Events are characterized by a unique version number and are uniquely identified by an event identifier assigned by the responsible or recording healthcare agent.

Events and modifications to events correspond to two different types of event-related operations:

- creation of an event when new information is added, and
- creation of a new version when information is modified.

Events can serve as reference points helping to form a view of the patient record and improve efficient access to patient data. They support the following views:

- *Single patient view*: patient-oriented (longitudinal view of patient encounters) or visit-oriented (access to a particular admission or ambulatory visit);
- *Multiple patient view*: location-oriented (in which patients are present at a given location) or provider-oriented (in which patients are currently assigned to a given provider).

Classes of Clinical Data: The User Point of View

Clinical data consist of general identifiers (patient identification data, healthcare professional identification data, etc.), pure health-related data, general data (Figure 6.2), and also modifiers and qualifiers (Figure 6.3).

Encounter element	Requirement
Basics	
Identification	Data about a patient that rarely change (e.g., name, date of birth, Social Security number)
Social circumstances	Terms that describe the patient's environment, social network
Clinical information	
Chief complaint (CC)	Should be captured in every note
History of present illness (HPI)	Symptoms reported by the patient or other observers through normal clinical listening and questioning describing the patient's health status. Includes the following elements: location, quality, severity, duration, timing, context, modifying factors, and associated signs and symptoms
Review of Systems (ROS)	Consists of constitutional symptoms (e.g., fever, weight loss)
	(continued on next page)

Figure 6.2: List of the most important information categories in electronic health records. Based partially on the headings framework [NHS 2001].

Encounter element	Requirement
	(continued from prior page)
Physical exam (PE)	Findings elicited by a physician during the physical examination
Risk factor (alerts)	Information that the healthcare professional needs to be aware of but that is not a problem or a diagnosis Include allergies, prostheses, implants (e.g., pacemacker), and warnings (e.g., on anticoagulants)
Diagnostic tests and treatments Objective *non-interpreted*	
Investigations and test results	Tests, measurements, and procedures to obtain further information about a patient's status elicited by a physician and the use of appropriate technologies (laboratory, radiology, etc.)
Treatments and interventions	Therapeutic actions to improve the health status. Immunizations, counseling, education
Medication	Ongoing and proposed prescription of drugs
Decision making Objective *interpreted*	
Assessment	Based on the interpretation of data, the assessment phase may cover the following: • (*Differential*) *diagnoses:* represent the hypotheses that potentially explain the data: labels for communication. Covers all relevant diseases, disorders, and syndromes. May be qualified by: priority, certainty, linkage, importance, severity, and complication • *Rationale for a selected plan*: activities that a clinician or team intend to perform at a future time • *Summary* of the patient's condition or course of illness • *Problem list*: clinical information items that need to be considered by the healthcare professional for further action. Problems cannot be isolated entirely from diagnoses and have an important role in the multidisciplinary approach • *Hospital discharge summary:* a crucial element in the electronic health record that is mostly reflected in the discharge letter sent to the GP or referring physician
Plan	
Contains	Future actions that have to be undertaken (treatment goals, actions planned to attain a goal, expected outcome or prognosis)
Provides	Simple means of informing health-care providers or oneself about items needing attention

Figure 6.2: *Continued.*

Subjective data include verbal data originating directly from the patient: patient's complaints, patient's symptoms, clinical history, allergies, drug history, and so on.

Qualifiers	Roles
• abnormality qualifier	• role for
• existence qualifier	- healthcare professional
• successfulness	- patient
• spatial qualifiers	- patient relative
- relative position	• role in healthcare process
- side (left, right)	• healthcare professional relationship
- position of patient	• position of healthcare professional
• **time-related qualifiers**	• subject of information
- life cycle: done, in process, planned	• dates
- occurrence status	- documenting
- potentiality	- awareness, diagnosis
- process status	- clinical events
- obsolescence	
- level of urgency: emergency, routine	
- timing marker	

Figure 6.3: The importance of qualifiers and roles within medical data.

Objective data include data originating from medical devices (lab analyses, CT, ECG, etc.), the results of tests and investigations, or physical examination.

After collecting the subjective and objective data, a hypothesis is made. A process of differential diagnosis is started, narrowing a list of possible causes of the symptoms that potentially explain the data collected so far. The rationale for making a differential diagnosis is the selection of an intervention plan. Afterward, a summary of the patient's condition or course of illness is provided.

Plans include future actions (diagnostic or therapeutic steps) that have to be undertaken.

Headings for Communicating Clinical Information

To enable physicians to arrange data to fit their personal preferences, the concept of communication headings is important. A heading is an annotation mechanism for combinations of health data contained in the EHR. As part of the work in ToMeLo [ToMeLo 1997] a tentative categorical structure extracted from a few medical record systems was presented in the position paper: "Headings for Communicating Clinical Information from the Personal Health Record." A list of the most relevant categories based on the headings framework was presented in "Headings for Communicating Clinical Information" defined by the National Health Services [NHS 2001]:

1. *Health characteristics* describing the state of a patient: investigations (tests results), diagnosis, history, physical examination (findings), family history, and social circumstances.
2. *Actions* that describe anything that can be done to or for a patient: clinical assessment, treatment, informing, communicating, and clinical administration.
3. *Time modifiers* correspond to health characteristics and actions that occurred, are ongoing, or need to be done. Definition guidance for time modifiers are past, present and plan and outlook (correspond to health characteristics that a clinician or team envisages for a patient or a citizen in the future). At present they have defined four types of outlook: goal, prognosis, outcome, and risk. Based on work in CENTC251 on temporal attributes, Figure 6.4 lists 13 temporal comparators. Empty cells indicate combinations not allowed.
4. *Role view headings* represent the view of a person involved in the healthcare process: reason for contact, problems, risk factor (alerts).

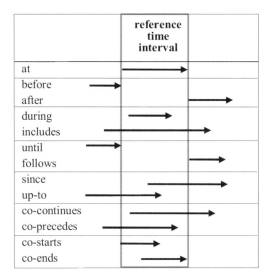

Figure 6.4: Reference time interval [CEN TC 251, prENV 12381].

Context

The *Concise Oxford Dictionary* defines context as a text preceding and following any particular passage, giving it a meaning fuller or more identifiable than if it were read in isolation.

In our society communication between two people is mostly verbal or written. Little attention has been paid to the accompanying contextual information such as severity, certainty, emotion, anxiety, hope, feeling, and other fuzzy values. Those attributes, although of much importance in a medical environment, are difficult to grasp in the spoken world but disappear nearly completely in the written world [Baud 1994].

The transmitter (source) communicates constrained information to the receiver who needs to unpack that information to try to rebuild the context in order to capture the semantics of information transfer (Figure 6.5). Likewise, health records store more than just subjective and objective patient data. They also store contextual information about medical events (patient's illness, examination, treatment, and so on) and the rationale justifying a particular action. Basically, this consists of descriptive information on those medical events and the relationships between them.

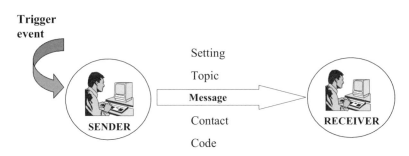

Figure 6.5: The seven constituents of communication.

To prevent the misinterpretation of data when it is communicated between two parties, the context must be preserved and stored. Since it is impossible to discuss the full scope of the issue of context, our discussion must be limited to the consideration of a relatively small number of areas in which progress can be made.

Examples of contextual areas are the source (originator) and location of information, the method of observation, the intent (or goal) of an action, and the expected receivers (the audience) [Degoulet 1989].

Health Records Structures

Time- and Source-Oriented Health Records

Countries differ in their legal and administrative policies about the healthcare record and the way information is organized. Health records can be structured in various ways: source-oriented, time-oriented (longitudinal), problem-oriented, and so on.

Paper records structure information in the same way as books and periodicals: hierarchical (e.g., table of contents), indexed in a one-dimensional space. The earliest medical records were organized in a *time-structured* way. They were real case "histories" [De Vries 1975].

Currently, most health records are *"time- and source-oriented"* (or information provider-oriented), and within each source category the information is time-sequenced. The health record is organized by specialty, each specialty possibly having a separate file. The physician updates the health record within different sections: observations, progress notes, prescriptions, requests for tests, and so on. The content of the record is heavily influenced by the corresponding medical specialty. The potential disadvantage lies in the fact that the synthetic part (e.g., the diagnosis discussion) may be neglected in favor of the analytical part (e.g., the physical examination and review of systems), hence neglecting problems not relevant for that specific medical specialty.

Problem-Oriented Health Records

As manual health records are often composed of chaotic narrative with seemingly unstructured components, Weed proposed in the 1960s an alternative to traditional time-oriented record keeping, the *problem-oriented health record* (POMR), structured around active and inactive problems [Weed 1968]. Weed also identified four major kinds of clinical data: subjective, objective, assessment and plan data (SOAP) as shown in Figure 6.6 [Weed 1969]. In this organization, three main parts constitute the structure of the record:

- The problem list designed to act as an index to easily view relevant parts related to one specific problem;
- Basic information containing patient demographic data and information that may be changed over time (location, marital status, employer, etc.); and
- Progress notes ordered in the SOAP format.

Abdominal pain	Hypertension	Type
Epigastric pain Awakes patient	Headaches	S
Normal examination	BP: 166/84 mm Hg Pulse: 88 Bodyweight 53 kg	O
Ulcus	Hypertension	A
Gastroduodenal endoscopy Diet	Beta-blocker 1/day Diet	P

Figure 6.6: POMR examples.

This SOAP categorization of data has been criticized due to the pejorative term (subjective data) used. Donnelly et al [Donnelly 1992] proposed using the term *history* for a narrative account, and *observations* covering the terms subjective and objective (HOAP) mentioned earlier.

The first two categories originate from the patient. The latter two are related to the physician. The structure of the POMR increases the readability of the health record by forcing the physician to adopt a systematic problem approach (Figure 6.7). Although there are a number of disadvantages inherent in this hierarchical treeing, such a model is suitable if there is independence between certain branches (problems) of the hierarchy, which is seldom the case. Hence the risk arises that information may be duplicated or even inconsistent (e.g., beta-blockers prescribed for one problem may have contra indications for another one).

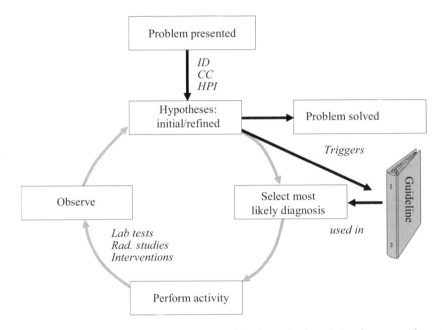

Figure 6.7: A schematic representation of the hypothetico-deductive reasoning of medical decision makers during collection and interpretation of medical data. This iterative process is repeated until a hypothesis is reached.

A *problem* is a finding or process that requires consideration for diagnostic evaluation or therapeutic intervention (Figure 6.8). As Weed explained, a problem could be anything: a sign, a symptom, an abnormality, a treatment, diagnosis, social complaints, or anything else that has been observed regarding the patient. However, a problem is not a superordinate concept. The problem must be able to develop and change without modifying the underlying observations. Related concepts include plans, which link events to problems or observations, and episodes, which group visits or periods of care together in ways that reflect the physician's understanding [Rector 1991].

The evolution of a person's health status is considered a succession of problems, reflected in a problem list giving rise to the possibility of a problem-oriented view of the EHR. The purpose of a problem list is to give the healthcare provider a tool to organize problem-oriented information. Problems are characterized as having a beginning and ending date. Other attributes of a problem are mentioned in Figure 6.9. Additionally, problems may be related to other problems (with relationships such as secondary-to, caused-by, and associated-with).

The definition of a problem is left to the authority of the supervising (or attending or treating) physician. When a problem is resolved, its status is switched from active to passive. Several problems can be created concurrently. Preferably problems are selected from a predefined problems list. These lists serve as the basis for the establishment of a protocol. The EHR system may display a list of currently active problems, objectives and goals. Medical activities that are a part of a plan can be reviewed in terms of their respective statuses. A complete history and physical write up includes an assessment. The assessment begins with the patient's problem list, and is followed by a listing of their possible causes with their differential diagnoses. The problem list contains the items known to be true (e.g., weight loss, fever, and chest pain).

Problem type	Description	Example
Diagnosis of x	The patient has a medical condition corresponding to a diagnosis based on recognized and explicit criteria	Hypertension
Chief complaint x	Currently hospitalized for diagnosis x	Hospitalization for congestive heart failure
History of x	The patient had x (diagnosis, procedure, etc.) in the past, and that fact should remain on the active problem list	Diagnosis: history of pulmonary tuberculosis Procedure: mitral valve replacement
Family history of x	Family history of diagnosis x	Family history of colon cancer
Certainty of x	The physician must rule out diagnosis x Diagnosis x is uncertain	Rule out myocardial infarction
Symptom/sign of x	The patient has symptom/sign x	Symptom of shortness of breath
Risk of x	The patient is at increased risk for diagnosis x	High risk of lung cancer
Take note of x	Medical or nonmedical condition of importance (e.g., wheelchair required)	

Figure 6.8: Various types of problems may occur. Previously inactivated problems can be reactivated.

Although the POMR concept is well accepted, its benefits have not been demonstrated and it is difficult to implement in complex practices [Salmon 1996, Wyatt 1994]. Few healthcare organizations have succeeded in implementing POMR for care delivery. The difficulties that have to be taken considered when introducing the POMR are:

- The growth and difficult maintainability of the list of problems. Problems can be in an active, resolved, or dormant state. Moreover, problems tend to arise and be resolved over a long period. They also change over time [Claus 1997].
- Lack of a clear definition of a "problem" just as there is a lack of a clear definition of a "disease" or a "diagnosis" [Tielemans 1998].
- The *vagueness* of problems often linked in a casual way, as expressed differently by several providers.
- The difficulty in assigning each finding to one of the problems stated in the problem list.
- Medical data may belong to more than one problem. Problems can be composed of other (sub)problems. For example, ischemic heart disease may have such sub-problems as angina, myocardial infarction, and ventricular failure, all of which need to be considered separately.

Attributes	Description	Examples
Common term	Shorthand terms for convenience	CHF (congestive heart failure)
Problem status	Active or inactive	
Temporal terms	Beginning and ending dates	
Physician	Treating Supervising Assisting	
Anatomic	Location	Head, neck, shoulder, upper extremity, thorax, abdomen, pelvis, knee, ankle, foot
Relative position	Laterality, situation	Right, middle, left anterior (ventral), middle posterior (dorsal), cephalic (upper)
Classification code	Classifying a diagnosis, surgical intervention	ICD-10, SNOMED, CPT
Severity indicator	Scoring for a specific disease, for categories of patients	Glasgow Coma Scale, ICU-APACHE III
Pathologic process	Describes disease process affecting the organ system	Fracture Neoplastic: benign, malignant
Etiology	Physical factors	Burn, impact, neoplastic, metabolic
Linkage identifier	Specifies relationships between problems and other events	Caused by, originated from

Figure 6.9: Attributes of a problem.

Results can be associated with clinical problems, by source, or chronologically. The linkage between problems and results may be explicitly defined.

Episode-Oriented Health Records

Health records can be organized around episodes. For example, information is related to a hospitalization period (reason for admission) or to a chronological set of activities during a closed series of healthcare sessions. The record is terminated with a final discharge note.

Solon et al. [Solon 1967] define an episode of care as "a series of temporally continuous health care services related to treatment of a given state of illness provided in response to a specific request by the patient or other relevant entity" (Figure 6.10). An "episode" is a situation where duration is considered highly relevant.

The diagnostic content of an episode of care has been largely debated in the literature. Some claim that a specific problem is not necessary for its existence. Others discuss whether an episode corresponds to a problem or if various problems must be contained by a single episode.

Although the usefulness of episodes of care has frequently been demonstrated, few healthcare organizations have succeeded in implementing episode-based structures for care delivery. Problems encountered were the definition of provider responsibility, determination of the end point of care, the capture of problems (which may change over time), and the aggregation of elemental data into workable "chunks" [Claus 1997].

In 1996 the Mayo Clinic in Rochester, whose traditional paper-based system has relied on a type of "episode of care" basis, adopted a new definition of care made available to more than 3000 EHR-capable workstations. The main idea was to assign each patient to an initial service and provider responsible for the opening of the episode. This primary provider would note the patient's problem episode information and initiate orders. Other providers might note additional problems and create additional orders. The primary provider registered the endpoint of the episode. However, if a patient subsequently reappeared, a new episode would be opened. Mayo episodes of care are defined as follows:

- non-overlapping periods of clinical care;
- begins with first service or test given to the patient;
- coordinated by a single "primary provider";
- completed by dismissal of care by the primary provider (including review of care and problem list and the explicit declaration of "dismissal");
- allows for multiple problems with focus on those problems currently being addressed;
- supports an integrated group practice model
    - multiple provider record management, and
    - multiple provider problems list management; and

• multiple author document management [Solon 1967, Weed 1969, Salmon 1996].

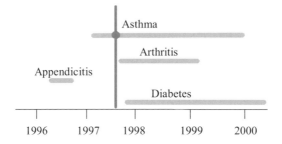

Figure 6.10: A timeline showing a single encounter versus episodes.

Pragmatic Medical Records

In the pragmatic record model proposed in 1989 by P. Degoulet, observations, actions or abstractions (i.e., concepts) are always considered in the context of their production [Degoulet 1989]. Five pragmatic (contextual) axes (S, T, O, R, and M) are considered indispensable for building a pragmatic model: the source of observation (or action), the event and Time of observation (or action), the observation or action objects and their interaction, the receiver, and the methods used (i.e., to produce an observation or an action) (Figure 6.11).

	Observation	Action	Abstraction
Example	SBP is 220 mm Hg	Furosemide 25 mg *bid*	Hypertension
Source	Physician = x	Physician = x	World Health Organization
Time interval and event	$[t_1 - t_1]$	$[t_1 - t_2]$	$[t_1 - t_2]$
Object(s) and their interactions	(O_1) Patient = y (O_2) SBP = 220 mm Hg (O_1) *has* (O_2)	(O_1) Patient = y (O_3) Furosemide = 25 mg *bid* (O_1) *is treated by* (O_3)	(O_4) Disease = Hypertension (O_5) Vascular disease = disease category $(O4)$ *is a* (O_5)
Receiver	To whom it may concern	To whom it may concern	Medical community
Method	Manual BP measurement	Medical prescription	SBP ≥ 160 or DBP ≥ 95 mm Hg

Figure 6.11: Abstractions, actions, and observations in the STORM pragmatic model. SBP: systolic blood pressure; DBP: diastolic blood pressure (adapted from [Degoulet 1989]).

Other pragmatic axes, such as the location (e.g., the place an observation was made or the location of an action) or the intention (i.e., the health goal such as the reduction of a risk factor or the prevention of a disease) can be included and implemented in an extended version of the model.

The source of information is always a key element of the context, since it partly or fully supports the act of interpretation. For a medical observation or action, the source can be a physician, nurse, patient, automatic device (e.g., a blood pressure monitor), or computer program like an expert system. For an abstraction (e.g., the concept of blood pressure or hypertension), the source can be an expert or a community of physicians.

Several concepts are associated with the time axis, including events or points in time, intervals, periodic time, and precedence (e.g., before, after). Points in time are represented as intervals with $t_1 = t_2$.

Objects are defined by the classes to which they belong, by their behavioral properties inherited from classes and superclasses, and by their links (e.g., *is a*, *has*, *caused by*, *treated by*, etc.) to other objects. The term *receiver* is applied in a broad sense. A receiver might be the addressee of a message, the patient to whom a drug is given, the community for which a concept is to be used (e.g., the medical community for the concept of hypertension), or a receptor in a biologic structure. Methods express the way in which the relationships between the source, the objects, and the receiver are obtained. For example, the method of blood pressure measurement might be auscultation, the automatic detection of sounds with a microphone, or a Doppler method. The method of recording a symptom might be a patient interview by a physician or a computer.

Health Record Component Architecture

An electronic health record architecture must be capable of structuring data and dealing with the data-intensive nature of medical applications. Healthcare information is *huge in volume*, keeps increasing, and is *multimedia in form*. Some entities of this health record are multi-user in nature (e.g., patient demographic data, lab results, and observations), while others are single-user but feature a highly complex structure (e.g., radiotherapy radiation schemes). Technical achievements on the software (graphical user interfaces and object-oriented techniques) and hardware levels (cheap storage and extensive computing power) provide new opportunities that have, in the past, conditioned existing electronic health record systems.

The EHR is a data-repository containing statements and facts about patients under treatment. It uses medical concepts supplied by a knowledge component (terminology server). The health record is the unifying instrument that integrates the large amounts of patient data originating from laboratories and radiology and other medical services. EHRs are collections of entries (observations, vital parameters, textual information, etc.) that accumulate chronologically and progressively as the medical history of the patient evolves over time. Observations can be composed of elementary or composite observations derived from observational concepts defined in a medical thesaurus. Because of the huge variety of information used, third normal Codd representations as found in classical relational database theory are not practical and are structured too rigidly for proper use in the design of electronic health record systems. There is a need for a more advanced flexible storage structure. Different possible approaches are canonical representation, tagged components, or object representation in triplets (object–attribute–value as used in conceptual graphs).

Two major approaches to the design of EHR architectures are emerging: the middleware or object-oriented conceptual scheme and the document-oriented approach [Takeda 2000].

Europe has launched various initiatives to define the architecture of an EHR. Two initiatives coincide at a certain point. One is the GEHR project (Good European Health Record) derived from an European Community (EC) research and development program in telematics [GEHR 1992]. The second arose from the EC standard committee CEN/TC251. The working group one (WG1) is devoted to building a standard for the EHR (Project Team PT011). The OO approach initially defined in GEHR has subsequently been revised in other projects such as Synapses [Synapses], EHCR SupA [EHCR], and CorbaMed [CORBAmed].

Another example of EHR architectures emerged in Internet environments through the use of the hypertext metaphor and XML as the technology for describing electronic documents. It gave birth to the document-oriented approach applied in the HL7 PRA project [HL7] and the Japanese MML project [Yoshihara 1998].

The logical constituents of the EHR repository are explained below. This explanation is based on the EHR CEN/TC251 prestandards prENV 12265 [CEN 1995] and prENV 13306 [CEN 2000]. The main constructs expressed in these pre standards are the *health record item* (HRI), and the *health record item complex* (HRIC) which are briefly explained hereafter.

Health Record Item

A HRI (health record component in prENV 13306) is the basic unit of health information within the EHR. It represents the finest level of granularity that remains meaningful as an entry in the record. It can be processed by means of basic operations such as add, move, and delete [Maskens 1993]. Record items hold data and are primarily composed of a name and a value. Examples of individual record items could contain the units, value, label of a measurement:

> measurement label—"albumin"
> measurement value—"6.9"
> measurement unit —"Mol/l"
> comment —"approved"

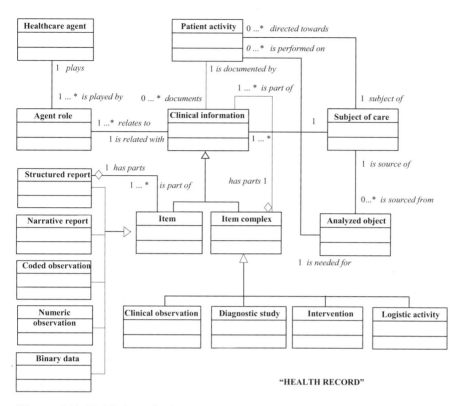

Figure 6.12: Unified Medical Language (UML) diagram of the medical record component. The care activity class originating from the act component generates clinical information. Clinical information corresponds respectively to the health record item and health record item complex.

Health Record Item Complex

An information element in a health record has a specific place and a specific composition dependent on the healthcare professional view. For example, some physicians prefer an anamnesis located at the beginning of the record, others might prefer to display it as a request or under another label. Therefore, the EHR will be built in such a way as to separate structure (know-how) and data (patient-related). Under the structure model, the layout and representations are independent and flexible.

A HRIC (selected component complex in prENV 13306) represents this logical structure of records (grouping record items and record item complexes). It is an abstract construct that has the basic properties required for the aggregation in the record. The root of the aggregation is the record itself. So the EHR itself will be regarded as a record item complex. A record item complex can belong to one of the following subtypes: an *original record item complex* or a *view record item complex*.

An *original record item complex* (original component complex in prENV 13306) represents the original record context for the information it contains and for the description of the grouping and ordering of subsidiary record items or record item complexes. For example, the blood pressure level as a record item complex contains two components record items, the systolic and the diastolic blood pressure.

A *view record item complex* is used for the description of the grouping and ordering of subsidiary record items or record item complexes, which are selected by criteria or by reference. The content shall be either

- one or more criteria for the selection of records, or
- one or more references to HRIs or HRI complexes as data are often presented in more than one part of a record.

Figure 6.12 shows a conceptual diagram partially based on the CEN/TC251 prENV 12265 prestandard. The clinical observation class can be further subtyped into clinical assessment, physical examination, and chief complaint. The diagnostic study class is a generalization of measurements done to obtain further information about a patient's health status and corresponds to the results of lab tests, radiology studies, ECG, EEG, and so on. Interventions group the outcome of actions performed by a healthcare agent to improve the health status of a patient and correspond to medication administered, immunizations given, surgery, radiotherapy, chemotherapy, and so on. Finally, logistical activities are done to support the clinical work, and include admittance, patient transfer, and certificate completion.

In conclusion, the recursive structure of an HRI complex allows the health record items to be assembled into completely flexible but valid structures, of which the largest collection would be the entire EHR itself.

Links with Other Components

To exploit the underlying concepts of HRIs and HRICs, the health record component must collaborate with other components, especially with the knowledge component that will be discussed in more detail in Chapter 7.

Within each medical domain, the knowledge component is responsible for the definition, content, and structure of the medical data. In the knowledge component three types of application agents characterized by complementary competencies are considered: a terminology part, a problem-solving part (inference engine), and an ontology part.

The ontology part defines the concepts and their relationships in the domain of discourse, and focuses on the semantic aspects aiming at global consistency. It consists in the example of Figure 6.13 of a semantic network with a direct cyclical graph to provide multiple and coexisting hierarchies.

The terminology part (controlled vocabulary) covers a semantical network of medical concepts that is language-independent in contrast with the classical enumerative classification of terms found in terminologies like ICD-9-CM or SNOMED.

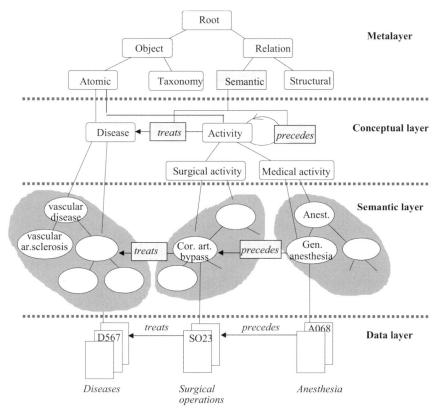

Figure 6.13: Taxonomy of medical concepts embedded in a semantic network.

Semantic networks are structures for representing knowledge and are composed of nodes and links (semantic relationships). The former represent concepts, the latter relationships between concepts, clarifying linguistic cases (agent, patient, recipient, etc.) or spatial temporal or logical connections. The semantic network is based on non associative medical concepts (semantic types) and associative (medical) concepts (relations). It operates at different stages of data input (control, validation) and output (active, passive reminders, help functions). In medicine, multiple inheritance occurs frequently (one concept that inherits properties from various ancestors).

Health Record Management

User Interface Component

The presentation component is responsible for the provision of a flexible way of displaying or capturing data through a graphical user interface (GUI). These adaptive user interfaces are essential for EHRs.

Information ergonomics deals with the design of presentation formats, visual conventions, data entry and presentation methods, and navigation through the system. Transferring patient records from paper to screen may have important consequences. Physicians are often reluctant to use IT technology. Their resistance is due to the fact that a lot of existing computerized tools are not properly designed. Otherwise why, if paper-based methods are less efficient, and if the benefits of IT systems outweigh the inconveniences, would doctors be reluctant to use them?

In 1988, Van Bemmel described the user interface as one of the most important challenges in medical informatics [Van Bemmel 1988]. In spite of these obstacles, little literature on designing effective user interfaces for clinical practice is available. Inconsistency, insufficient navigation control, and difficulties in accessing important procedures are often the case in today's systems.

Three goals should serve as a guide in proper user-interface design [Nygren 1996]:

1. *Learning.* It must be easy for the user to learn how to use the interface, and the learning time must be short. Intuitive user navigation, configurable screens adapted to each clinician's practice patterns, short response times, and replicated document (metaphor) as workspace are some of the methods that can be used to achieve that goal.
2. *Efficiency.* The interface must provide added efficiency in daily work or fast response times adapted to the user's daily practice.
3. *Excellence.* The interface must provide excellence or the potential to reduce the probability of error [Helander 1988].

The risk of information overload is only marginal, but the risk of cognitive tunnel vision due to too little simultaneous data is much greater.

Strategies of Clinical Data Entry at the Point of Care

Clinical practice focuses on patient care, whereas clinical information systems focus on the record of that care. Much of the information captured at the point of service in health records must be captured by healthcare agents who are authors and users as well. The vocabulary used in medical notes is highly dependant upon the medical speciality. Medical texts sidestep the normal rules of expression of any natural language (especially from the syntactical point of view), and tend to use nominal phrases and a restricted number of significant verbs. It often features conjunctive enumerations of features, separated by commas, used to explain signs, symptoms, and numerical results. It is not unusual to find syntactical errors [Alpay 93]. But even in the case of semantic ambiguities, the medical context helps to adjust the errors that are made.

Direct entry by healthcare professionals is important for obtaining timely, precise information. As stressed before, the most critical challenge in the acceptance and implementation of a computerized health record is the capturing and authentication of data gathered by physicians. How can we be assured that physicians' observation notes are correctly and completely entered into the computer? This can only be achieved by minimizing the time and optimizing the incentives for physicians. As G. Hripcsak [Hripcsak 1995] wrote, "A patient and a provider engage in a complex encounter involving the patient's concerns, symptoms, history; the physical exam; and the provider's assessment, plan, actions and results. Unfortunately, our computer systems capture a mere shadow of the encounter." We should keep in mind that data—whether stored centrally or distributed—has to be collected for a certain purpose, otherwise the data are not valuable.

So by succeeding in capturing the encounter, we can improve care in several ways. Six criteria are important for information gathering [Rector 1996] completeness, accuracy, availability, speed, user, and patient acceptability. The issue is how to enter relevant clinical data. Several options are available.

Free Text

Free text is perhaps the most widely known and used approach today in capturing patient data. It provides the user with unlimited freedom of expression at the expense of uniformity and consistency. Approaches to capture the patient encounter include

- scanning paper notes as free text;
- voice entry as a free text; and
- voice recognition, which is the conversion of spoken words into computer text. Speech is first digitized and then matched against a dictionary of coded waveforms. The matches are then converted into text as if the words were typed on the keyboard.

Transcription

One estimates transcription costs at around 15 cents/line or between $2 and $3/page corresponding to an average of $3.50/report. The reports are not immediately available due to final verification, and this delay may often lead to degrading practice efficiency. One study of 4871 radiology reports from the Brigham and Women's Hospital (Boston) demonstrated that 33.8% of the reports required post-transcription editing by radiologists prior to signature. At teaching institutions, report signature often causes additional delays, as the reports have been dictated by trainees or assistant physicians, and have not yet been reviewed, edited, and signed by the senior physician who is legally responsible for the report. This review is typically performed in batch version, further delaying the final report.

Transcription errors and missing or incorrect information may lead to unnecessary treatment or testing, or can cause a risk of complications or morbidity for the patient.

Finally, since the semantic content is neither stored nor indexed, a text report is not useful for decision support. It only permits text-based searches that are time-consuming and characterized by low response times.

Structured Reporting

Instead of free text, structured data entry (form based) based on an underlying descriptive knowledge model is being pursued as an alternative approach. The patient's entire care delivery process—medical history, symptoms, physical examinations, differential diagnosis, problems—is registered as discrete events using a structured data-capture approach rather than as strings of free text.

The success of structured report systems is intrinsically coupled with the use of the appropriate medical terms. Again, the wide adoption of structured reporting systems necessitates lexicons for all medical disciplines. Therefore, physicians who use structured report systems must familiarize themselves with preferred terms for findings. For unfamiliar findings, a physician must initiate a search for the proper term, rather than entering the concept as free text or using an approximate synonym. For radiologists, for example, structured reporting systems (like some speech recognition systems) may cause the radiologist to spend more time checking the report as it is produced and less time examining the images thus affecting the accuracy. As a result, what should be a production task becomes a search task [RSNA 2000].

The representation methods that must be looked at and may be used jointly are formatted screens, hierarchical linked lists, and text screens of free texts.

We must be aware that the usefulness of data for advanced functions, such as intelligent queries, decision support systems, quality assurance, and research, increases with the degree to which they are structured. Free narrative text is difficult to control and difficult to analyze and to aggregate for analytical purposes. On the other hand, the only access facility available with text files is running a search on (pre)-indexed keywords corresponding to the content of the document, or character string alternatives that are far from ideal and possibly inaccurate in terms of the information supplied.

Coded Entry

The entry of codes based on a coding or classification scheme may be the approach that results in the most information. Users must be familiar with coding schemes beforehand to accurately reflect the real situation. On the other hand, coded entry systems may sometimes hamper the productivity of, and limit the freedom of expression of, users. It is therefore necessary for the proper combination of text-oriented, unstructured systems and coded data entry to be found according to the formalization of the domain of application (Figure 6.14). Existing coding systems, although relatively advanced, are often considered to be too rigid and too succinct to support clinical care and to capture clinical details. A single coding system serving the needs for all medical departments is not realistic, but the definition of a core model of the semantics of medical concepts is feasible. This is one of the objectives of the GALEN project [Rector 1998].

Coding is in essence a reduction process. The more structure and coding are embedded in the EHR

- the less user-friendly the behavior of the system and the more difficult it will be to overcome the resistance of physicians to capturing the information of physicians by voice, by menu selection, by keyboard, and/or pointing devices; and

- the easier it is to achieve the detailed analysis of information included in the health record for

  - outcome analysis, providing information on morbidity, mortality, case mix, severity, comorbidity, and so on;

  - utilizing review studies on personnel and at the facility management level;

  - trend analysis studies, evaluating developments in medical care delivered (medical treatment profile, administered drug-profile, etc.), patient referral demographic area, and so on; and

  - quality of care evaluation including clinical competence, and appropriateness and effectiveness of medical care delivered to the patient.

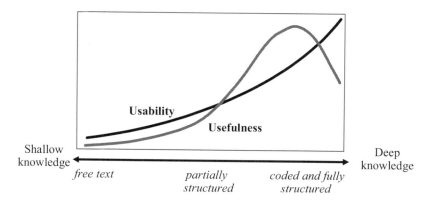
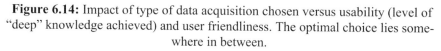

Figure 6.14: Impact of type of data acquisition chosen versus usability (level of "deep" knowledge achieved) and user friendliness. The optimal choice lies somewhere in between.

On the other hand, the semantic content of (coded) data is dependent on the precision with which it is coded, and its utility decays proportionally over time due to the lack of detail and context information. A good coding system should provide features to define the context explicitly. Therefore, the use of free text is much richer than codes.

Natural language processing (NLP), although still not widely available, could be used for extracting codes and classification. In the foreseeable future, the use of NLP modules in well-defined domains will allow mapping free text into identifiable codes. According to G.C. Chute: "NLP is the grail of systems integrators and workstation developers accepting natural language from care providers, transparently mapping these observations using a language-independent conceptual scheme, manipulating the interlingua objects to pose germane conceptual queries to appropriate knowledge sources, and provide clinically relevant feedback to the care provider derived from certified authority" [Chute 94].

Presentation for Reading and Interpretation

The problem does not end with the storage and retrieval of information in the format in which it was registered [Tang 2001]. There is a requirement for the same information to be available in different formats depending on the desired context and preferences of the clinician. Some medical departments will register additional specific information on a patient for internal use, which may be required only by that department when carrying out activities (e.g., radiation details for that patient). Therefore, information must be filtered in the EHR according to the profile of the health professional user retrieving the record. In many cases, parts of the medical data on patients may be held electronically on different departmental computer systems within the hospital.

The essence of a good EHR system is the ability to retrieve the data needed—no more, no less. It is counterproductive to display more data than necessary. Displaying overviews of data where the system requests more actions if the user desires detailed information makes looking up the information faster and more efficient. This stresses the importance of a workflow management component that offers the ability to "prefetch" some large volume data such as medical images.

It is remarkable that in a system's development life cycle relatively more time is spent on designing the layout for data entry than on viewing forms (i.e., what information should be presented and how). In most cases, the layout for data entry and for reading need not be the same. However, data are of no value if they are not used and the way one reads data can either lead to the probability of arriving at erroneous conclusions or the possibility of achieving excellence [Nygren 1996].

User Interface Design Guidelines

The following guidelines should be taken into consideration:
- Use large screens (minimum 17 inches): the complexity of physicians' tasks means they are often confronted with a variety of different types of information that must be displayed simultaneously.

- Carefully design the layout of the overview (summary) screen to allow for the quantity of data that needs to be viewed in parallel. Display only relevant information and remember that the first view should attempt to provide a rich overview of information about the patient (allergies, risk factors, outstanding examinations, actual medication, etc.) and not a menu of available functions. It should be possible to recognize a case prior to further actions.
- Try to avoid the "windows overconsumption" syndrome where diverse data groups are presented in separate windows.
- As it must be possible to rapidly page through multiple-page textual information, provide features (hypertext approach) to intuitively page through a complete record.
- Take into account page size as one of the factors that affects reading speed on the screen [Reisel 1997, Creed 1988, de Bruijn 1992]. The smaller the page the slower the reading. Type font does not have a significant effect on reading speed [Frenckner 1990].
- Respect the chart presentation format often used on ward units and especially in ICUs. Data need to be viewed in different time scales and in different decision-making situations. Remember the risk of information overload is only marginal, but the risk of cognitive tunnel vision due to too little simultaneous data is much greater.

Summary and Conclusions

Electronic health records will not substantially change the format of the classical paper-based medical record. Although technology is available and strong efforts are under way everywhere to make the transition from a paper record to a complete EHR feasible, in most organizations this will not be the case in the very near future. The main problems are human, organizational and financial.

The Web technology offers novel challenges and opportunities. Users will impose higher requirements resulting in EHRs based on networked interactive hypermedia documents, which are different in one crucial aspect: hypertext links allow users to access a single page with no preamble.

An electronic health record not only is a tool for gathering and representing data, but also must reflect the static (representation of data) and dynamic character of medical care as well (i.e., what actions are going on, what interventions are planned, scheduled for a patient, etc.). In fact an EHR can be found at the intersection of the static and dynamic spheres of health care. The passive health records of today will change into active objects.

The intelligent coaching features added to this health record will give rise to standardized vocabularies and messaging systems.

The structure of an electronic health record can be viewed in four different ways

- a longitudinal life-long record;
- a problem-oriented record that documents patient problems and diagnoses initiated by a start date and finalized by an end date;
- an episode-based record in which care episodes are defined by end and start dates; and
- a pragmatic record in which observations, actions, or abstractions are always considered in the context of their production.

In conclusion, we can summarize the "gold standard" attributes for the computer-based health record as mentioned by the Institute of Medicine (IOM) [Dick 1995]. An electronic health record system has to offer the following features:

- a problem list;
- the ability to measure the patient's health status and functional levels;
- a tool to document clinical reasoning and rationale;
- a longitudinal view that provides timely linkages with other patient records;
- guaranteed confidentiality, privacy, and audit trails;
- continuous access for authorized users;
- support for simultaneous multiple user views;
- direct data entry by physicians;
- support for practitioners in measuring or managing costs and improving quality; and
- flexibility in supporting existing or evolving needs of clinical specialities.

References

[Alpay 93] Alpay L, Baud R, J-R Scherrer. Representing semantical knowledge of medical texts for natural language processing. In: *AIM-CEN European Workshop on the Medical Record*. Brussels: March 31–April 2, 1993; pp. 298–303.

[Bainbridge 1996] Bainbridge M, Salmon P, Rappaport A, Hayes G, Williams J, Teasdale S. *The Problem Oriented Medical Record—Just a Little More Structure to Help the World go Round?* Clinical Computing Special Interest Group (CLICSIG) of the PHCSG. http://www.ncl.ac.uk/~nphcare/PHCSG/conference/camb96/mikey.htm, 1996.

[Baud 1994] Baud R, Rassinoux A, Wagner J, Lovis C, Juge C, Scherrer J. Representing Clinical Narratives. *Sowa Conceptual Graphs IMIA WG 6 - Working Conferences,* Geneva, (May 29–June 1), 1994.

[Bishop 1991] Bishop CW. A new format for the medical record. *MD Computing.* 1991; 8(4): 208–215.

[CEN 1995] CEN/TC251. *PrENV 12265. Electronic Healthcare Record Architecture.* July 1995. [http://www.centx251.org].

[CEN 2000] CEN/TC251. *PrENV 13606-1. Electronic Healthcare Record Communication.* May 2000. [http://www.centx251.org].

[Chute 94] Chute GC, Cesnik B, Van Bemmel JH. Medical data and knowledge management by integrated medical workstations. Summary and recommendations. *Int J Bio-Med Comput.* 1994; 34: 175–183.

[Claus 1997] Claus PL, Carpenter PC, Chute CG, Mohr DN, Gibbons PS. Clinical care management and workflow by episodes. *Proc AMIA Annu Fall Symp.* 1997; p. 91–95.

[CORBAmed] CORBAmed. http://www.omg.org/homepages/corbamed/.

[Creed 1988] Creed A, Dennis I, Newstead S. Effect of display-format on proof-reading with VDUs. *Behav Information Technol.* 1988; 7: 467–478.

[De Brota 1994] De Brota DJ. In front of us. *Int J Bio-Med Comput.*1994; 34: 131–135.

[De Bruijn 1992] de Bruijn D. The influence of screen size and text layout on the study of text. *Behav Inform Technol.* 1992; 11: 71–78.

[Degoulet 1989] Degoulet P, Jean FC. The need for pragmatic database models. In: Scherrer JR, Côté R, Mandil S, eds. *Computerized Natural Medical Language Processing for Knowledge Engineering.* Amsterdam: North Holland, 1989; pp. 157–67.

[De Moor 1994] De Moor GJE. The future and the Impact of Telematics for Healthcare. *Proc Workshop European Health Care Record Architecture,* Brussels, 1994.

[De Vries 1975] De Vries R. Useful elements of POMR [report of experience]. *Med Rec.* 1975; 16(6): 13–17.

[Dick 2000] Dick R, Andrew WF. Explosive growth in CPRs: evaluation criteria needed. *Healthcare Informatics.* April 1995; 110–114.

[Donnelly 1992] Donnelly WJ, Hines E, Brauner DJ. Why SOAP is bad for the medical record. *Arch Intern Med.* 1992; 152: 481–484.

[EHCR] EHCR Support Action Project: http://www.chime.ucl.ac.uk/HealthI/EHCR-SupA/.

[Frenckner 1990] Frenckner K. Legibility of continuous text on computer screens —a guide to the literature. *Report no. 25 from IP* Lab, Royal Institute of Technology, Stockholm, 1990.

[GEHR 1992] *GEHR Projects.* Requirements —deliverables 4–9: http://www.chime.ucl.ac.uk/HealthI/GEHR/GEHR. Foundation: http://www.gehr.org/, 1992.

[GEHR 1993] *The Good European Health Record AIM Project* 2014. Deliverable 1–6, 1993.

[Helander 1988] Helander M, ed. *Handbook of Human-Computer Interaction.* Amsterdam: North Holland, Elsevier Science, 1988.

[HL7 1999] HL7 SGML/XML SIG: Patient Record Architecture/Kona Proposal. http://www.mcis.duke.edu/standards/HL7/committees/sgml/white-Papers/Prap/, 1999.

[Holman 1994] Holman BL, Aliabadi P, Silverman SG, Weissman BN, Rudolph LE, Tener EF. Medical impact of unedited preliminary radiology reports. *Radiology* 1994; 191(2): 519–521.

[Hripcsak 1995] Hripcsak G. Call for participation. *IMIA Spring Congress,* 1995.

[Iakovidis 1998] Iakovidis I. Toward personal health record: current situation, obstacles and trends in implementation of electronic healthcare record in Europe. *Int J Medical Inform* 1998; 52: 105–115.

[Johnson 1997] Johnson SB, Terre P, Khenina A. Generic database design for patient management information. *Proc AMIA Annu Fall Symp.* 1997; 22–26.

[Kuperman 1990] Kuperman GJ, Garoner RN. The impact of the HELP computer system on the LDS hospital paper medical record. *Proc 14th Annu Symp Comput Appl Med Care.* 1990; 673–677.

[Maskens 1993] Maskens AP. *GEHR General Syntax and Semantics: Interim Description.* Brussels: AIM Office, Deliverable 10, 1993.

[McDonald 1988] McDonald CJ, Tierney WM. Computer stored medical records: their future role in medical practice. *JAMA.* 1988; 259: 3433–3340.

[Medialogic] http/www.medialogic.com/products/implementing/ whitepapers/ dl_struclo2.doc.

[NHS 2000] *NHS Information Authority.* Headings for communicating clinical information draft information standard headings framework version 2. Final Draft, March 2000.

[Nygren 1996] Nygren E, Allard A, Lind M. Skilled users interpretation of visual displays. Report no 63/96 from Center for Human-Computer Studies. Uppsala, Sweden: Uppsala University, submitted, 1996.

[Rector 1991] Rector AL, Nowlan WA, Kay S. Foundations for an electronic medical record. *Methods Inform Med.* 1991; 30–38.

[Rector 1994] Rector AL, Soloman WD, Nowlan WA, Rush TW. *A Terminology Server for Medical Language and Medical Information Systems.* Geneva: IMIA WG 6-Working Conferences, 1994.

[Rector 1995] Rector AL, Medical-concept models and medical records: an approach based on GALEN and PEN&PAD. *J Am Med Inform Assoc.* 1995; 2(1): 19–35.

[Rector 1996] Rector AL. Computer-based patient records. In: Van Bemmel JH, McGray AT, eds. *Yearbook of Medical Informatics.* Stuttgart: 1996; 195–198.

[Rector 1998] Rector A, Rossi A, Consorti MF, Zanstra P. Practical development of re-usable terminologies: GALEN-IN-USE and the GALEN Organisation. *Int J Med Inf.* 1998; 48(1-3): 71–84.

[Reisel 1997] Reisel JF, Schneiderman B. Is bigger better? The effects of display size on program reading. In: Salvendy G ed. *Social, Ergonomic and Stress Aspects of Work with Computers.* Elsevier Science, 1997; 113–122.

[RSNA 2000] RSNA Radiology Society of North America. Efficient Multimedia Report Creation SR System 9502 NT-I, 2000.

[Salmon 1996] Salmon P, Rappaport A, Bainbridge M, Hayes G, Williams J. Taking the problems oriented medical record forward. *Proc AMIA Annu Fall Symp.* 1996; 463–467.

[Solon 1967] Solon JA, Feeney JJ, Jones, SH, Rigg RD, Sheps G. Delineating episodes of medical care. *Am J Public Health.* 1967; 57: 401–408.

[Synapses] Synapses Project: http://www.cs.tcd.ie/synapses/public/.

[Takeda 2000] Takeda H, Matsumura Y, Kuwata S, Nakano H, Sakomoto N, Yamamoto R. Architecture for networked electronic patient record systems. *Int J Med Informatics.* 2000; 60: 161–167.

[Tang 2001] Tang PC, McDonald CJ. Computer-Based Patient-Record Systems. In: Shortliffe EH, Perreault LE eds. *Medical Informatics. Computer Applications in Health Care and Biomedicine.* Reading, Massachusetts: Addison Wesley, 1990; 327–358.

[Tielemans 1998] Tielemans L. *Het medisch dossier.* Uitgaven VUB. Brussels,1998.

[ToMeLo 1997] Details on ToMeLo can be found at: http://www.ehm.kun.nl/tomelo. ToMeLo Workshop; Paris CNIT La Defense, 1997.

[Tuttle 1994] Tuttle MS, Stuart JN. The role of the UMLS in storing and sharing across systems. *Int J Bio-Med Comput.*1994; 34: 207–237.

[van Bemmel 1988] van Bemmel JH. Medical data, information and knowledge. *Methods Inform Med.* 1988; 27: 109–110.

[Weed 1968a] Weed LL. Medicals record that guide and teach. *N Engl J Med.* 1968; 278: 593–599, 652–657.

[Weed 1968b] Weed LL. *Medical Records, Medical Education and Patient Care. The Problem Oriented Record as a Basic Tool.* Cleveland: Case Western Reserve University Press, 1968.

[Weed 1969] Weed LL. *Medical Records, Medical Education and Patient Care.* Cleveland: Case Western University Press, 1969.

[Weed 1971] Weed LL. The POMR as a basic tool in medical education, patient care and clinical research. *Ann Clin Res.* 1971; 3: 131–134.

[Whiting-O'Keefe 1988] Whiting-O'Keefe QE, Whiting A, Henke J. The store clinical information system. *MD-Comput.* 1988; 5(5): 8–21.

[Wyatt 1994] Wyatt JC. Clinical data systems. *Lancet.* 1994; 344: 1543–1546.

[Yoshihara 1998] Yoshihara H. Development of the electronic health record in Japan. *Int J Med Inf.* 1998; 49: 53–58.

7

The Knowledge Component

The main goal in health practice is to correctly interpret patient data and then to make sound medical decisions. Professionals rely on academic/scientific knowledge accessible from the literature and on more practical expertise derived from their experience with previous cases. The decision process is complex because of a rapidly changing and expanding nature of all these forms of knowledge. Indirect indicators of this complexity are the continuous expansion of the specialized terminologies and the exploding volume of knowledge sources, either in paper or electronic format (e.g., full text electronic journals).

Knowledge-based systems (KBSs) cover a large variety of computer applications that manage general or specialized knowledge. They include software tools as diverse as terminology managers, expert systems, and case-based reasoning engines.

In contrast with more traditional processing systems that were focused on quantitative and numerical analysis of data, knowledge-based technology often concentrates on qualitative analysis and symbolic reasoning techniques [Haas 1986]. In theory KBSs do not suffer from human weaknesses. They are permanently and ubiquitously available. They have nearly unlimited capacities and are not emotionally conditioned. They can solve complex situations efficiently and constitute the natural complement to traditional database management systems as shown in Figure 7.1 [Grimson 1988]. For instance, an expert system might use the patient's history from a conventional hospital information system database to predict a diagnosis or plan a medication strategy.

In practice, KBSs have given rise to misunderstandings and premature expectations.[1] Despite the tremendous amount of energy that has been devoted to this area by key research groups since 1970, most expert systems developed for the healthcare environment never left the research institution or were limited to the education domain [Healthfield 1994, Lincoln 1991]. Because of their high resource consumption and complexity, the systems that

---

[1.] For example, expectations that could be drawn from Stanley Kubrick's *2001: A Space Odyssey* (1968) or, Steven Spielberg's *Artificial Intelligence* (2001).

run are frequently implemented on separate computer systems with little or no integration into the underlying clinical production system.

	Data-based systems	**Knowledge-based systems**
Representations and use of	Data	Data and knowledge
Efficiency	Efficient management of large volumes of data Requires storage capacities	Processor consuming
Used for	Medical data for patient management and statistical studies	Medical knowledge for decision making and explanations
Models	Data models - flat files - hierarchical - network - relational - object-oriented	Knowledge models - production rules - frames - semantic networks - logic - neural nets
Processes	Record keeping Repetitive actions Algorithms	Heuristic classification Deductive, inductive, abductive reasoning Genetic algorithms

Figure 7.1: Knowledge-based versus data-based systems in medicine.

Indeed, barriers to the development of expert systems were clearly recognized and discussed in the early 1980s. They include the difficulties in formalizing medical knowledge, in finding the right experts and agreeing on consensual items of knowledge, and in maintaining existing knowledge bases or evaluating running systems.

This chapter discusses the methodologic approaches and components that can make a clinical information system support sound medical decision making.

Conceptual Specifications

Types of Knowledge

Knowledge refers to the kinds of information that can improve the efficiency and effectiveness of a problem solver [Hayes-Roth 1994]. There are four major types of knowledge: structural, beliefs, heuristics, and causal relationships.

Structural knowledge is the easiest type of knowledge to formalize. They correspond to a "what is" form of knowledge.

Examples:

- A heart has two ventricles.
- The aorta divides into the two iliac arteries.

Beliefs express plausible propositions. They correspond to more subjective knowledge to which certainty indicators can be associated.

Heuristics are rules of thumb that express methods of applying judgment in situations for which valid algorithms generally do not exist. Simple heuristics are step-by-step procedures to follow. They correspond to a "how-to" form of knowledge.

Examples:

- If the patient has a high temperature and chills, stop the blood transfusion immediately.

- If an epileptic patient has partial seizures and carbamazepine does not sufficiently control the seizures then, sodium valproate may be tried.

More complex heuristics express strategies that address a given situation.

Example:

- Do not prescribe drugs whose combination is strongly contraindicated.

Causal and *temporal relationships* are common in the health domain. Medical signs or symptoms frequently follow a specific chronology. Causal relationships add a cause/relationship factor to a temporal series of events.

Examples:

- Increased demand for oxygen increases the heart rate.

- Inflammation causes an increase in the temperature of the surrounding tissues.

Knowledge Representation Formalisms

The question of knowledge representation, which was at the center of artificial intelligence (AI) discussions in the 1970s, remains crucial to the design of any KBS. Conceptual design in this field is based on the understanding of what knowledge representation is and how it can be used to build an efficient decision support system (DSS) [Davis 1993, Shortliffe 1993].

Figure 7.2 illustrates, from a rough analysis of the table of contents of the three textbooks in artificial intelligence, how the field of knowledge representation has evolved in 25-year period to become a central issue. Several inference mechanisms can be associated with each representation formalism. Knowledge begins with the observation of the world and the attempt to organize objects and facts. Knowledge elements are the conceptual constructs created by observers (e.g., human beings) on the observed world. A concept is an intentional representation of a class of objects. Concepts are considered the building blocks for our understanding of cognition and the construction of mental models.

Knowledge representation	Winston [1984]	Winston [1992]	Negnevitsky [2001]
Semantic nets and frames (No. of pages and %)	37 (31%)	92 (34%)	34 (15%)
Production rules (No. of pages and %)	37 (31%)	60 (22%)	30 (13%)
Logic (No. of pages and %)	44 (38%)	40 (15%)	
Neural nets (No. of pages and %)		61 (22%)	54 (23%)
Probability networks (No. of pages and %)		18 (7%)	32 (14%)
Fuzzy logic and reasoning			42 (18%)
Genetic algorithms			40 (17%)
Total (No. of pages and %)	118 (100%)	271 (100%)	

Figure 7.2: Knowledge representation covering (and associated reasoning mechanisms) in three textbooks on artificial intelligence.

With one problem as a base, several knowledge representations need to be discussed and often combined to build a sound KBS. An evaluation of the decisions proposed by the KBS might lead to refining or reformulating the knowledge hypotheses in a knowledge decision loop (Figure 7.3).

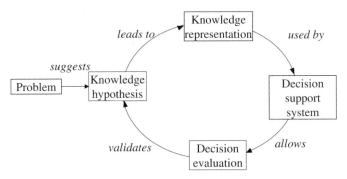

Figure 7.3: The knowledge–decision loop [Degoulet 1995].

Semantic Networks

In a semantic network, the knowledge base consists of a collection of nodes connected by arcs. The nodes represent concepts, whereas arcs give the relations (i.e., the semantic links) between them. The *is-a* link (e.g., is an instance of) and the *has-a* link are the two key relationships found in most semantic networks. They can be extended to more complex relationships like *causes*, *inhibits*, *stimulates* to represent pathologic or physiologic knowledge. Through *is-a* links, concepts inherit the properties of their parents or ancestors.

Semantic networks constitute the key formalism for building ontologies of medical terms and terminology servers. They are not adapted to express procedural knowledge or heuristics. Examples of KBS applications based on semantic networks are CADUCEUS, CASNET and MEDES. Figure 7.4 gives an example of a semantic network for representing physiologic knowledge.

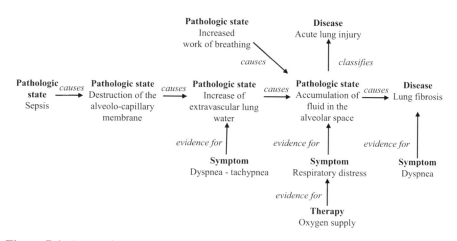

Figure 7.4: A causal network in the domain of acute respiratory distress syndrome, a pathology that often occurs in intensive care units. Nodes represent "states" and links represent "causal relationships" between those states.

Frames or Structured Objects

A frame is a generalized formalism introduced by M. Minsky to represent knowledge about objects that uses slots [Minsky 1975]. Frames are also referred to in the literature as scripts, schemes, prototypes, or structured objects.

Both declarative and procedural knowledge may be stored in the slots of a frame to produce specific behaviors. Frames may be linked by their slot values in *is-a* links or subtyping relationships. Rules can be represented as a specific type of arc.

Figure 7.5 gives an example of a hypothetical knowledge base on drugs that is built on a frame-based knowledge representation with subclasses and instances. The APTINE and INDERAL frames are two instances of the BETA BLOCKER frame.

In the frame-based QMR system the disease frame has weighted links to various signs, symptoms, and other diseases [Rennels 1987]. *Evoking strength* weights reflect the likelihood that the disease is present when a certain symptom is observed: 0 means that the symptom is nonspecific and 5 means that the disease is the only cause of the symptom. Frequency weights indicate how likely the disease is to give rise to a particular symptom. A value

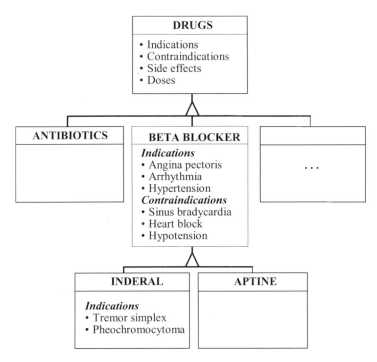

Figure 7.5: A frame-based knowledge representation.

of 1 means it does so rarely, whereas 5 means it does so in almost every case (Figure 7.6).

Frame name: Tularemia Symptoms and signs	Evoking strength	Frequency
Fever	0	5
Skin lesion: culture *Francisella tularensis*	5	4
Lymph node enlarged	1	4
Skin ulcer	1	4
ECG sinusal tachycardia	0	4
Tularensis skin test positive	4	3
Exposure to rabbits, rodents, small mammals	2	3
Tick bite recent history	2	3
Headache severe	1	3
Can cause		
Pyrogenic shock	1	2
Acute appendicitis	1	1
Predisposes to		
Endocarditis acute infection, left heart	1	1

Figure 7.6: The QMR frame system. Adapted from "Advanced Computing for Medicine," by Glenn D. Rennels and Edward H. Shortliffe. Copyright © October 1987 by *Scientific American*, Inc. All rights reserved.

Production Rules

Rules are formulated as if/then clauses. If the condition is true or has reached a certain degree of validity, then the conclusion or action is activated. The general form of a rule is as follows:

IF <condition> THEN <conclusion/action>.

Figure 7.7 gives an example of a rule in the MYCIN expert system.

RULE 156

IF:

1. The site of the culture is blood, and
2. The Gram stain of the organism is negative, and
3. The morphology of the organism is rod, and
4. The portal of entry of the organism is urine, and
5. The patient has not undergone a genitourinary manipulative procedure, and
6. Cystitis is not a problem for which the patient has been treated

THEN: *There is suggestive evidence (0.6) that the identity of the organism is E. coli.*

Figure 7.7: A rule in the MYCIN expert system. Adapted with kind permission from Bruce G. Buchanan and Edward H. Shortliffe.

The inference engine of a rule-based system checks whether all conditions are true for a specified problem.

Limitations of this representation formalism have been widely debated [Talmon 90]. First, rules do not represent the basic or deep knowledge of a domain, but merely compiled, shallow knowledge. This limits the amount of explanation that a rule-based system can give. Second, its weakness in viewing a problem from different perspectives narrows its problem-solving capabilities. Third, it is often difficult to specify when a certain rule is valid. Although a rule may state a generally valid association between the condition and conclusion part, there might be many exceptional situations in which the rule is not valid. One need simply glance at the indications and contraindications for prescribing a drug. The list of contraindications is often impressive, while the indication for giving a drug is most often one simple sentence. Hence there is a need for a method to describe the context in which the rule is valid.

Logic

The basis of *propositional logic* is established by combining propositions or axioms applying Boolean algebra with logical connectors such as

OR   disjunction
AND   conjunction
NOT
IMPLICATES

IS EQUIVALENT WITH

Predicate logic, also known as first-order logic, is an extension of propositional logic, which introduces the concepts of variables, quantifiers, and functions. Formal language can be used to formulate axioms, which are statements describing the universe of discourse.

For example, the sentence "If an epileptic patient has partial seizures and carbamazepine does not sufficiently control the seizures, then sodium valproate may be tried" will be expressed as follows:

> DIAGNOSIS   (*epilepsy, X*)
> EPILEPSY TYPE   (*partial seizures, X*)
> DRUG PRESCRIBED (*carbamazepine, X*)
> SEIZURE STATUS   (*controlled, X*)
> DRUG TO BE TRIED (*sodium valproate, X*)

X is used as a variable that is bound to the patient identification during the problem-solving process.

Other Representation Systems

As shown in Figure 7.2, multiple representation formalisms have been proposed in addition to the previously described ones. In the neural network approach, units do not tend to represent complex concepts. They correspond to relatively simple features or microfeatures that are active subsystems of a complex system. The information is passed among the units not by symbols but by numbers, and the interpretation of the processing is done not in terms of messages being sent but of the identification of the active states.

The fuzzy logic approach tries to mimic the ability of the human mind to effectively employ modes of reasoning that are approximate rather than exact. In the last decade acyclic-directed graphs have been used to represent uncertain relationships, including belief networks and influence diagrams.

Inferences and Problem-Solving Techniques

Reasoning Techniques

Deductive reasoning is based on the principle of logical implication. It allows inferring conclusions with a degree of certainty based on the degree of certainty of the premises. In general, deductive reasoning provides the possibility of switching from a more general to a more particular case (hence, deriving new facts).

Example:

> Every man is mortal; Socrates is a man.
> Hence, Socrates is mortal (**modus ponens**).

Inductive reasoning provides the capability of switching from a particular to a more general case. It produces inferences that are valid to a certain degree of probability or credibility.

Example:

A, B, C,... are men and are mortal.
Hence, man *X* is mortal.

Abductive reasoning derives from the experimental approach. A number of observations are considered. The researchers or the computerized systems look for relationships between those observations, such as a causal relationship. These hypotheses may indicate the selection of an existing law or the definition of a new one.

Heuristic classification is a method of solving problems that uses rules to aggregate data into categories, map categories into enumerated solution categories, and select a solution set from the solution categories. For example, given data in the form of medical symptoms such as runny nose and teary and itchy eyes, rules may be used to classify the data into a problem category called allergy. Additional rules may be used to map allergy problems to a solution category such as antihistaminic drugs. Refinement rules are then applied to select one specific antihistaminic drug.

Inference Engines

An inference engine in a KBS specifies the logical process by which new facts and beliefs are derived from preexisting facts or beliefs [Haynes 1990]. It also contains the control strategy that orders the search for an inferential solution. An inference engine is basically a pattern matcher. It searches the knowledge base to find a structure that is in agreement with the known and derived facts of the problem to be solved. When such a structure is identified, the specified action is taken. The choice of the type of inference depends on the nature of the problem to be solved, the knowledge hypotheses, and the knowledge representation model(s) selected.

In production systems, *forward* or *data-driven reasoning* techniques start from known facts or data and determine what conclusions can be reached from these facts using a set of production rules. *Backward reasoning* or *goal-directed inferencing* identifies a hypothetical conclusion (e.g., the suspected diagnosis is gastric ulcer) and verifies whether this conclusion can be proposed because the facts defined in the condition parts of a rule are present.

Blackboard systems use multiple independent knowledge sources to analyze different aspects of a complex problem. Each knowledge source contributes its information to the common working memory, referred to as the blackboard. A master control program continually examines the blackboard and orders the agenda of what to do next. Blackboard architectures compose solutions from component subsolutions, each of which may be generated or notified by its own knowledge sources or mini-expert systems.

Constraints are kinds of meta-rules that can be used to maintain consistency in knowledge bases (e.g., temporal reasoning or updating probabilities). In general, a constraint has a premise establishing a relationship between objects. When this relationship holds, the constraint allows deducing knowledge on other objects from the knowledge. Constraint propagation has similarities with rule inferencing. When the value of a constraint's premise is known, unknown values are inferred as far as possible. Then the constraint is fulfilled, a contradiction has to be resolved (e.g., by eliminating a wrong fact), or the constraint may be fulfilled later, when further values are known [Tusch 1990].

Decision Analysis

In decision analysis, a decision tree diagrammatically represents the clinical alternatives. By convention:

- Square boxes define decision nodes (i.e., actions or alternatives).
- A chance node is represented by a circle, from which several alternatives are drawn. Probability estimates are assigned to each branch.
- Every chance node is characterized by a number called the expected value. It is the value that is expected on the average for a specified chance event or decision.
- At the end of each branch, the outcome of the corresponding strategy is calculated (utility values).

In performing a decision analysis, several steps have to be taken: after designing the decision tree and assigning probabilities and outcome utilities, expected values in every chance node have to be calculated. Subsequently, the alternative with the highest expected value is chosen and finally the decision-making process ends with a sensitivity analysis.

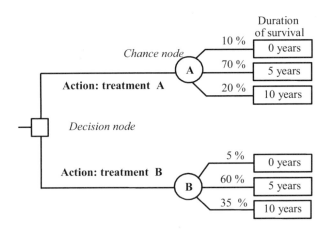

Figure 7.8: Example of a decision tree representation of surgical intervention given two different treatments.

The decision criterion can be the duration or quality of life after treatment. This is defined as the *utility* and represents the value of a specific outcome to a decision-maker. An example of a decision tree is presented in Figure 7.8 with the following calculations:

Expected survival for treatment A
$$= (10\% \times 0) + (70\% \times 5) + (20\% \times 10)$$
Expected survival for treatment B
$$= (5\% \times 0) + (60\% \times 5) + (35\% \times 10) = 6.5 \text{ years}$$

Ontologies and Terminology Servers

To cope with a diversity of medical applications and the specific information they use, the creation and maintenance of controlled terminologies and coding systems remain a major challenge for medical informatics specialists [Sittig 1994]. Three kinds of information need to be specified: the precise definition and description of concepts, the criteria for classifying concepts into hierarchies, and the criteria for determining when two concepts are equivalent [Cimino 1989].

A *domain ontology* defines the representation vocabulary for a shared domain of discourse (e.g., classes, relations, functions). Problem-solving situations relate mostly to two kinds of ontologies: taxonomic and causal [Miller 1982, Van der Lei 1994].

- In a *taxonomic ontology* concepts (e.g., diseases) are defined as, or are associated with, a cluster of attributes (e.g., patient's manifestations) without cause-effect relationships.
- In a *causal ontology* (Figure 7.4) links between concepts represent causal or temporal relations. Causal ontologies may be represented by network behavior and functional and/or temporal models.

Although the standardization of medical language and terminology is a major concern, no single clinical terminology is yet in widespread use. Clinical terminologies need to support integration with clinical software and the conversion to existing reporting and epidemiologic coding schemes such as ICD-9-CM, CPT4, or SNOMED. Concept-oriented terminologies share a knowledge-based approach to term representation and make use of constructs such as semantic networks or conceptual graphs to provide explicit relationships among terms.

It is remarkable to see that a number of commercial vendors have chosen not to use standard terminologies but favor either systems developed in-house, or commercial interfaces such as those of Purkinje's MEDCINTM. On the other hand, standards committees such as HL7, LOINC, and DICOM have also developed their own special purpose terminologies.

Figure 7.9 illustrates the sources of medical concepts most commonly used to build controlled terminologies.

In his paper entitled "Clinical Terminology: Why Is It So Hard?" Rector gives 10 reasons why the development of terminology software is difficult [Rector 2001]:

1. "The scale and the multiplicity of activities, tasks, and users it is expected to serve is vast.
2. Conflicts between the needs of users and the requirements for rigorously developed software must be reconciled.
3. The complexity of clinical pragmatics-support for practical use for data entry, browsing, and retrieval and the need for testing the pragmatics of terminologies implemented in software.
4. Separating language and concept representation is difficult and has often been inadequate.
5. Pragmatic clinical conventions often do not conform to general logical or linguistic paradigms.
6. Both defining formalisms for clinical concept representation and populating them with clinical knowledge or "ontologies" are hard—and their difficulty has often been underestimated.
7. Determining and achieving the appropriate level of clinical consensus is hard and requires that the terminology be open-ended and allow local tailoring.
8. The structure idiosyncrasies of existing conventional coding and classification systems must be addressed.
9. The terminology must be coordinated and coherent with medical record and messaging models and standards.
10. Change must be managed, and it must be managed without corrupting information already recorded in medical records."

Terminology domain	Available sources of concepts
Sign, symptoms	Read Code, SNOMED RT, NANDA
Diagnoses	ICD-9-CM, ICD-10
Acts (laboratory, radiology)	CPT 4, ICD-9-CM, LOINC, NGAP, SNOMED International
Drugs	NDC, WHO Drug Dictionary
General classification and nomenclatures	MeSH, SNOMED-RT, UMLS

Figure 7.9: Available sources of concepts. SNOMED RT—Systematized Nomenclature of Human and Veterinary Medicine; NANDA—North American Nursing Diagnosis Association; ICD—International Classification of Diseases; CPT4—Current Procedures and Terminology; LOINC—Logical Observation Identifier Names and Codes; NDC—National Drug Codes; MeSH—Medical Subject Headings; UMLS—Unified Medical Language System.

As the sophistication of controlled medical terminologies has evolved from simple code-name-hierarchy arrangements into rich knowledge-based representations of medical concepts, the simple word processors used in the past to create and maintain those simple terminologies are insufficient. More sophisticated terminology tools often grouped under the broader term of *terminology servers* are required for maintenance and use. They include browsers that allow users to navigate through the terminology and complex searching and manipulation functions made available through well-defined application programming interfaces (APIs).

The UMLS metathesaurus and the SNOMED-RT nomenclatures are often proposed for inclusion into terminology servers due to their broad coverage. Significant examples of terminology servers are the VOSER vocabulary server to support the terminology needs of the HELP system at the Latter Saint Days (LDS) Hospital in Salt Lake City [Rocha 1994], the server for the GALEN project [Rector 1995], and the Medical Entities Dictionary (MED) used at Presbyterian Hospital in New York [Cimino 1989, 1994]. MED is a frame-based semantic network, in which each concept has a number of named slots with values that may be literal values or pointers to other MED concepts. It currently contains over 67,000 concepts, with terms drawn from those used in laboratory, pharmacy, radiology, and billing systems. It includes 206,000 synonyms, 100,000 hierarchical relations, 167,000 other semantic relations, and 139,000 mappings to other terminologies, including the UMLS, ICD-9-CM, and LOINC codes [Cimino 2001].

Given the broad interest in terminology servers, the Object Management Group (OMG) published a request for proposals for the drafting of specifications for Lexicon Query Services [OMG 1997]. Chute et al simplified this to a set of server requirements and identified nine desiderata for clinical terminology servers that would be used for data entry by clinicians: word normalization, word completion, target terminology specification, spelling correction, lexical matching, term completion, semantic locality, term composition, and term decomposition [Chute 1999].

Architectural Frameworks

Architectural frameworks for knowledge-based systems incorporate the following components or subcomponents (Figure 7.10): a knowledge acquisition tool, a terminology server, an inference and control engine, a working data set (problem instance), and a data acquisition interface [Lanzola 1993]. They are also likely to contain an explanation module to help justify the decisions or recommendations presented to the end-users.

EON is a good example of a knowledge engineering environment. It was developed at Stanford University and provides tools to manage knowledge structures (domain ontology, eligibility criteria, abstraction definitions, guideline algorithms, revision rules, and a temporal query language), to make inferences, and to provide explanations [Musen 1996]. Based on patient data fed from a database with a specified temporal database manager or directly from user input, the appropriate recommendations based on the specific expertise are generated.

Clinical Decision Support Systems

Historical Background

As shown in Figure 7.11, the earliest decision support systems were developed in the 1970s and 1980s with the idea of supplementing or even replacing medical experts in domains such as blood infections (MYCIN), renal disorders (PIP), ophthalmology (IRIS), or more general internal medicine (INTERNIST). At the end of the 1980s, as happened in other areas as well, people realized that decision support systems could survive only if they could

- focus on limited problems in narrow domains, and
- fit to the medical user instead of fitting the physician to the decision support system through a true integration with the underlying clinical information system,

assist the physician instead of replacing him. The user interaction had to change from the Greek oracle mode of conversation to a close physician-computer system symbiosis [Miller 1990].

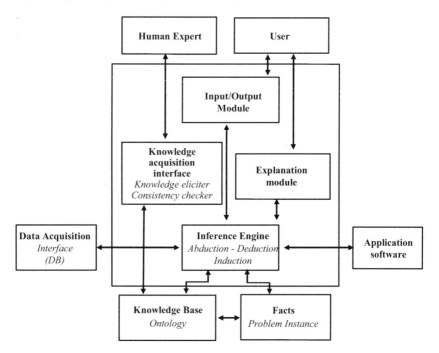

Figure 7.10: Components of a knowledge-based system.

Scope of Intervention

Decision support systems (DSSs) cover a large variety of computer programs that use clinical data and medical knowledge to perform one or more of the following tasks: serving as a tool for information management, helping healthcare workers focus attention, or giving advice in the form of a patient-specific consultation [Miller 1994].

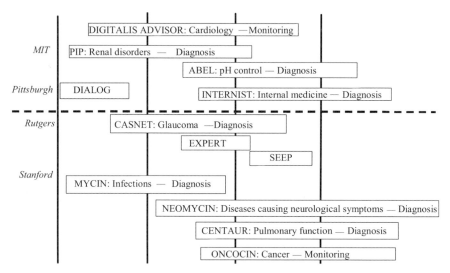

Figure 7.11: First general example of medical expert systems.

Simple alerts and reminders are the easiest form of support that a DSS can provide. They address, for example, the indication of abnormal values (e.g., a low potassium value) or the search for a drug contraindication or adverse drug interactions.

Clinical pathways describe a sequence of tasks such as the procedures that need to be conducted in conjunction with a given activity. This allows a care delivery system to better standardize medical practice. The scope of clinical pathways is useful when the medical situation is relatively simple, but the pathways are limited in their ability to support exceptions or decisions that go beyond the routine.

Protocols are precisely specified procedures that incorporate strict criteria for executing tasks and making decisions. A radiotherapy schedule for a specific tumor is an example of a protocol. A typical protocol consists of eligibility criteria, a sequence of tasks, which may be specified in the form of a flowchart, and conditions that would require a patient to be removed from the protocol.

Guidelines provide a description of clinical best practice, which is intended to be interpreted by the healthcare professional according to the patient's needs and related clinical conditions. Guidelines provide a general structure for defining tasks that may involve deciding between alternative treatments that may run concurrently, and interactions with other guidelines.

Problem-solving components perform well-defined tasks, typically to suggest a specific clinical approach or to support higher-level functions such as a combination of reminders, alerts, protocols, and guidelines. For example, medical researchers investigating breast cancer may have discovered statistical relationships between some of the determinants of survival following surgical removal of a tumor. So they create an application in which the user inputs values for age, menopausal status, estrogens receptor status, S-phase fraction, and so on, and the application outputs the likelihood of disease-free survival following the removal of a local tumor. The core of such an application is a predictive model that is packaged as a problem-solving component. Another example of a problem-solving component takes as input a standard clinical protocol description and relevant patient data and generates as output the qualitative likelihood that a patient is eligible for the given protocol.

Mode of Intervention

Passive systems await the user's input. They are defined in the literature as *interpretation systems* or *consultation systems*. Interpretation systems automatically provide information on request by the physician (e.g., the interpretation of an ECG). Consultation systems operate in an interactive dialogue with the clinical user. An early example of a consulting system is MYCIN, in which diagnostic advice is returned after the user manually enters patient information in response to a number of questions generated by the system [Shortliffe 1976]. Another example is Proto-VIEW [Vissers 1995], a protocol processing system supporting physicians in the emergency ward. With this system the user retrieves knowledge and navigates through protocols.

In an *active system,* the interaction with the DSS is direct and done automatically. Examples are *alerting systems* (e.g., the HELP system [Cannon 1980]) that generate reminders when certain activities are ordered (e.g., the search for a drug–drug or drug–lab interaction in a provider order entry system). They require access to the patient's entire clinical data. *Critiquing systems* generate case-specific advice or critiques for the user based on information on the patient status and strategy or objectives proposed for the patient (therapeutic or investigational) by the physician. An early example is the ATTENDING system developed at the University of Yale, to provide critiques for a patient on anesthesia or a antihypertensive program [Miller 1986]. Autonomous active systems have been embarked on intelligent monitoring environments. They can react to the storage of unusual clinical data in a clinical database (e.g., the change of vital patient parameters).

Another approach to categorizing DSSs is to base them on the time of interaction. *Real-time* DSSs (or event-based DSSs) are triggered by real- time events. *Prospective* DSSs analyze historical data to anticipate future events. Applications are found in care plan management, diagnostic support, and drug management (reminders, contraindications). *Retrospective* DSSs known in management literature as *executive information systems* (EISs) operate on historical aggregated data supported by data warehousing and data mining procedures.

All DSSs can be extended with an educational component and offer a teaching mode to the user. This is often a key factor in their clinical acceptance [Teach 1981].

Computer-Encoded Guidelines

Knowledge Sharing and Reuse

As the scope of medical knowledge is extensive by nature and the acquisition and maintenance of knowledge a time-consuming process, knowledge must be shared and reused. Following Musen's definition, knowledge sharing is the use of a given knowledge base at other sites or in different software environments [Musen 1993]. Moreover, knowledge is not fixed forever and must be continuously adapted. Those changes can be classified as follows:

- Modifications that change the structure of knowledge. Knowledge related to diagnosis and diseases are essentially structural.
- Modifications that focus on the factual part of the knowledge related to protocols and therapeutics, which is easier to achieve than the former.

Knowledge that is reused comes from existing KBSs or problem-solving methods; it is then used in significantly different contexts. Reuse of knowledge is an important issue in improving the knowledge acquisition process and in achieving cumulative growth. The components that can leverage knowledge reuse include the following [Musen 1993]:

- reusable ontologies (i.e., describing formal description of objects and their relationships);
- reusable terminology servers;
- a common inference syntax (e.g., Arden or GLIF syntax);
- reusable problem-solving methods;
- reusable tasks: every KB system executes at least one task; and
- reusable knowledge servers: KB systems must operate on a set of symbols that have precise and invariant meanings.

Knowledge bases must support clinical practice in general and institution-related knowledge specifically. The main concern when sharing knowledge modules between different healthcare organizations are the following:

- Institution-specific parts, such as

  - the different medical terminologies resulting in semantic mismatches; and

  - mapping of database queries to local databases. For example the Arden Syntax—a data driven DSS—isolates institution-specific parts of the database queries within a curly brackets notation ({...}).

• Technical aspects of trigger mechanisms and communication with the database.

The following subsection describes several standardization efforts to foster sharing and reuse of knowledge bases in the domain of guidelines.

Toward the Standardization of Electronic Guidelines

Clinical practice guidelines have been defined as "systematically developed statements to assist practitioner and patient decisions about appropriate healthcare for specific clinical circumstances" [Field 1990]. Integrating computer guidelines seamlessly requires that the clinical workstation display and activate the guidelines relevant to the current patient context and allow the user to select the required orders to be launched as part of the patient order entry system. Tu and Musen have identified five principal tasks that computerized guidelines (and, of course, guideline representation methods) should be capable of supporting [Tu 2000]:

• making decisions;

• sequencing actions;

• setting goals (e.g., specific patient states) to be achieved;

• interpreting data; and

• refining actions (e.g., breaking up into subcomponents).

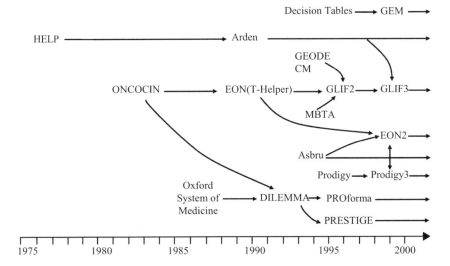

Figure 7.12: Historical illustration of the development of guideline modeling methods. Adapted from P.L. Elkin [2000].

Although clinical practice guidelines (CPGs) are well accepted, current experiences show a high diversity of modeling and implementation approaches (Figure 7.12). Some of them are briefly discussed below.

Medical Logic Modules and the Arden Syntax

The Arden Syntax—a rule-based approach for representing medical decision rules—was defined in 1989 as a standard format for medical knowledge representation in terms of *medical logic modules* (MLMs). Each MLM contains three parts: maintenance, library, and knowledge. The maintenance and library parts provide contextual information for the MLM, such as the title, author, version, creation date, and so on. The library part gives explanatory information about the MLM. The knowledge part is divided into four slots:

- The *data slot* couples the MLM with a patient database. The purpose is to define local variables used in the rest of the MLM. Within the data slot, the institution-specific portions are placed in mapping clauses so that the institution-specific part does not interfere with the MLM syntax.

- The *logic slot* contains clauses to be executed when the MLM is triggered. The logic slot uses data about the patient obtained from the data slot, manipulates the data, tests some conditions, and decides whether or not to execute the action slot.

- The *action slot* contains the action(s) to be carried out. Typical actions include sending a message to a healthcare provider, returning a result to a calling MLM, and evoking other MLMs.

- The *evoke slot* describes the conditions defined in the database tables that trigger a MLM. A MLM may be triggered by any of the following situations:

   - the occurrence of some event;

   - a time delay after an event;

   - periodically after an event; and

   - through a direct call from another MLM or a program.

The implementation of a medical decision support system based on the Arden syntax knowledge representation results in the realization of a data-driven decision support system. An event occurring in a medical database triggers one or more MLMs. An event (change in patient data) contains a trigger and a medical expression. The basic trigger types are insert, update, and delete. An MLM needs input data from one or more databases.

The input data are necessary to perform logic manipulations and to transmit results or messages to a certain destination if the logic concludes that the condition is "true." A MLM-based DSS engine has four main tasks to be executed in the following order:

- When will the MLM be executed (logic slot)?
- Which MLM will be executed (evoke slot)?
- How should data retrieval be handled (data slot)?
- How should the MLM actions, if any, be performed (action slots)?

The Arden Syntax reduces the risk of divergences between knowledge representation systems but does addresses the unified mapping between this knowledge formalism and local thesauri. Hence it requires local customizing. A study conducted by Pryor and Hripcsak [Pryor 1993] between the Columbia-Presbyterian Medical Center in New York and the Latter Saint Days (LDS) hospital in Utah showed that data base queries are the biggest challenge due to the differences within the local vocabularies. Again a major problem is the smooth connection of input data from one or more institution-specific file sources to the DSS engine (MLM). Either the data system delivers the data or data retrieval is executed from the MLMs.

The Intermed Guideline Interchange Format (GLIF)

Complex clinical guidelines require high-level control mechanisms. With the goal of reuse of clinical guidelines and the use software across institutions, the Intermed group, a consortium of Harvard, Columbia, Stanford, and other institutions, created the InterMed Common Guideline Model and Guideline Interchange Format (GLIF) to address the issue [Ohno-Machado 1998].

Version 2 of GLIF models guidelines as a flowchart of structured steps, representing clinical actions and decisions. GLIF3, which supports computer-based execution of guidelines, extends GLIF2 constructs and provides a more formal definition of decision criteria, action specifications, and patient data [Peleg 2000]. GLIF3 enables guideline encoding at three levels: a conceptual flowchart, a computable specification that can be verified for logical consistency and completeness, and an achievable specification that can be incorporated into existing clinical information systems.

GLIF specifications consist of the GLIF model and the GLIF syntax. The GLIF model is an object-oriented model that consists of classes, attributes, and the relationships among them (Figure 7.13). The syntax defines the format of the text file that contains the encoding.

The guideline intention describes the purpose of the guideline, currently encoded as narrative text. It includes eligibility criteria (a set of criterion objects) and didactics (including bibliographic citations or references to URL). Other classes in GLIF also allow the optional inclusion of external didactic information. Guideline steps cover action, conditional, branch, and synchronization steps. An action step is a class used for modeling actions to be performed in the patient care process. An action step may name a sub-guideline. Each action step contains exactly one action specification and one pointer to the next step in the guideline. A conditional step may link any guideline step to any other guideline step. A conditional step contains a condition that may be evaluated as true or false. Branch steps direct flow to multiple guideline steps. Synchronization steps allow modeling of multiple simultaneous paths through the guideline (Figure 7.13).

The Knowledge Interchange Format (KIF)

The Knowledge Interchange Format (KIF) is a very expressive language developed for the interchange of knowledge [Genesereth 1994].

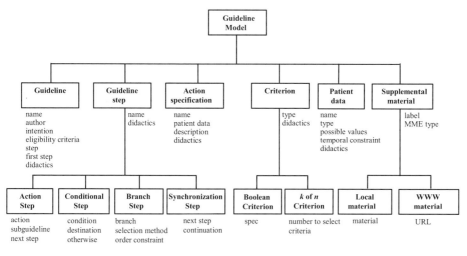

Figure 7.13: GLIF classes and attributes. *k* of *n* indicates *k* criteria from a total of *n* criteria. Adapted from "The Guideline Interchange Format: a model for representing guidelines," Ohno-Machado et al. Copyright © by JAMIA. 1998; 5(4) 357–372.

- It has declarative semantics because the meaning of expressions in the representation can be understood without appeal to an interpreter for manipulating the expressions.
- It is logically comprehensive because it provides for the expression of arbitrary sentences in the first-order predicate calculus.
- It provides for the representation of knowledge.
- It provides for the representation of non monotonic reasoning rules.
- It provides for the definition of objects, functions, and relations.

Other Approaches

Figure 7.14 illustrates the diversity of the modeling approaches.

ASBRU is an intention-based (i.e., goal-based) formal representation language for modeling guidelines developed by the ASGAARD project. An authoring tool converting text or HTML guidelines into XML and then into Asbru is currently under development.

Guideline Elements Model (GEM) is an XML-based mark-up model for guideline documents [Shiffman 2000].

GUIDE workflow involves the coordinated execution of multiple tasks performed by different agents, either human or technologic.

In Europe a cooperative effort resulted in the Prestige project, which represents guidelines as a structured set of subprojects [Gordon 1999]. The conceptual model originated from the DILEMMA (protocol knowledge representation), NUCLEUS (formerly known as RICHE, activity management), and GALEN (concept representation and terminology) projects.

The Prodigy KBS (Prescribing RatiOnally with Decision Support In General–Practice studY) includes a guideline-based decision-support system built on the EON model and designed to assist general practitioners in the United Kingdom [Sugden 1999].

EON [Musen 1996] is a component-based representation system containing knowledge structures. Using patient data fed from a database or from user input, recommendations are generated based on the specific guideline.

Prodigy is a guideline-based decision-support system built on the EON model and designed to assist general practitioners in the United Kingdom [Sugden 1999].

PROforma is a formal knowledge representation language for writing, publishing, and executing clinical guidelines [Fox 1998].

Models	Asbru	GEM	GLIF	EON	PROforma	Prodigy	Prestige
Algorithmic	Yes	Not prima-rily	Yes	Yes	Not primarily	Yes	Not prima-rily
Subguideline support	Yes	No	Yes	Yes	Yes	Yes	Yes
Supports decision criteria	Yes	Yes	Yes	Yes	Yes	Yes	Yes
Intentions and goals support	Yes	No	Through subguide-lines	Yes	Yes	No	No
Ranking of options supported	No	Yes	Yes	Yes	Yes	Yes	Yes
Temporal abstractions supported	Yes	No	No	Yes	No	No	No
Explicitly models patient preferences	No	No	No	No	No	No	No

Figure 7.14: Comparison between different guideline models. Adapted from Elkin [2000].

Knowledge-Based System Integration

Integration with Daily Clinical Practice

A major goal of knowledge-based systems is to be useful to health professionals. Therefore, they must be integrated into health professionals' daily practice. The consequence is that knowledge-based systems should not be used in isolation but should be integrated with the other software components that have been described in the previous chapters (e.g., the patient record or the resource component). Also, these systems should aim at providing global task support instead of creating separate systems (e.g., for diagnosis, treatment, and patient management) [Van der Lei 1994].

From the medical record point of view, three problems need to be resolved:

- a possible semantic mismatch between items in the KBS and the data model;
- a possible mismatch between item values at different sites (e.g., a normal value of sodium may be 120 to 140 mg/ml in lab X and 130 to 150 mg/ml in lab Y); and
- specification of the mapping process of data into symbolic values through

  - simple calculations, e.g., today − birthday → age .

  - symbolic mapping, e.g., $Na \geq 155$ mEq → hypernatremia .

  - inference mechanisms, e.g., physiologic value → pathologic state .

These aspects again underscore two issues in KBS integration:

- The need and importance of implementing EMR systems (*history, symptoms, signs, findings*) and to extend them with "rich" information produced by the KBS (interpretations of findings, statements concerning diagnoses, indications of treatment) [Lanzola 1993].
- The need for developing standardized ontologies of medical concepts. If the terminology of clinicians varies from place to place, a knowledge-based system is potentially useless and may be even dangerous [Barahona 1994a].

From the user point of view, it is important to fit the DSS to user needs instead of doing the reverse. End-user requirements need to be translated into functional, ergonomic, and psycho-cognitive constraints.

Although physicians were considered as the main users of DSSs, nurses, healthcare managers, and patients could also benefit from these systems. Nurses can benefit from DSSs in their daily activities: scheduling of health-care activities by automatic generation of healthcare management plans, intelligent information retrieval, and documentation. Healthcare managers could use KB technology to model the healthcare system by extracting information from aggregated data.

Integration with Clinical Protocols

In spite of the fact that most medical DSSs in the past have focused on diagnostic support, there is a growing consensus among medical users that determining the exact diagnosis is not the only goal of designing a DSS. Diagnoses are in fact working diagnoses on which a series of further subsequent actions—defined in clinical protocols—are based [Lanzola 1993]. Therefore, the use of clinical protocols (for nurses and physicians) is becoming more and more important.

First, the implementation of a protocol proves that a consensus has been reached among healthcare professionals. Moreover, the patient benefits from this type of care, considered and judged by a group of healthcare providers as the best and most efficient manner of handling patient problems. Also nurses benefit due to the fact that these protocols can clearly be documented in on-line textbooks. As the execution of a protocol may involve scheduling different activities in a number of medical departments, each related to different constraints, DSSs could offer support during the planning process to achieve optimal resource planning with reduced clerical time.

Second, once defined, these protocols are the basis for patient care plans and clinical studies when the outcome of patients treated with a specific protocol for a specific problem is compared to other groups, thus indicating the most appropriate protocol to be used.

Third, protocols that are clearly defined, and structured and composed of reusable diagnostic and therapeutic objects, are in fact already the basis for a KBS, and they improve in this way the knowledge acquisition process, reducing the gap between the knowledge engineer and the health professionals.

Integration with Patient Record Management Systems

To prevent the frustration of manually reentering data already available in computerized form, three approaches to solve this problem can be followed:

- enhancing an existing record management system with deductive capabilities (deductive database);
- coupling an existing record management system with an existing expert system (ES) tool (database–AI coupling); and
- extending an AI programming language with database management capabilities (enhanced AI systems).

Loosely coupled systems might result in excessive data traffic and query processing overhead, and the consistency between the two engines is not guaranteed, as there is no synchronization mechanism between them. One of the arguments for loose coupling between KBS and database management systems (DBMS) is that these are two substantially different technologic domains. Product developers of both domains pursue distinct aims, and extending one technology to incorporate aspects of the other might not be so easy. For example, how can we incorporate the features for concurrent access and protection into a tightly coupled system originally based on an AI system?

In the long run, the tight coupling strategy might be the preferred choice. This strategy executes database calls dynamically during the evaluation of a query. However, two major difficulties have to be solved when using this strategy:

- the complexity of queries, which can be higher than in conventional database applications, and
- the huge amount of database calls generated every time the knowledge base requires new facts.

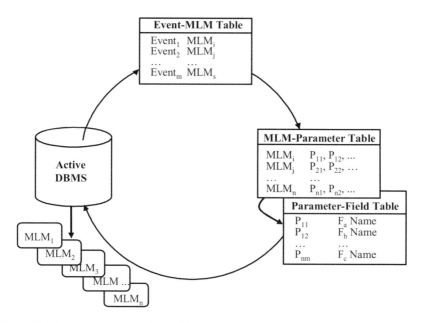

Figure 7.15: System mechanism with an active DBMS. The basic system components to connect database field names and MLM parameters are the event table, the MLM-parameter table, and the parameter-field table.

The following example illustrates the integration problem with the use of MLM-based DSS. Three approaches can be discussed:

- An *active* database sending trigger messages (to trigger the MLM) to the DSS engine when the data are stored or modified in the database, and transferring input data to the DSS (MLM) concurrently (Figure 7.15).
- The use of a *temporary storage* [Hongying 1995] where modified or inserted data is temporarily kept and the DSS engine triggers the DSS (MLM) afterward and transfers the MLM input data directly to the MLM (Figure 7.16).
- A separate *polling (monitoring) program* functioning as an external database monitor (e.g., in the case of a relational database management system (RDBMS) without active capabilities), which checks the database changes on a regular basis. When an MLM event is found, the DSS engine selects input data and triggers the MLM for further actions with the corresponding input data.

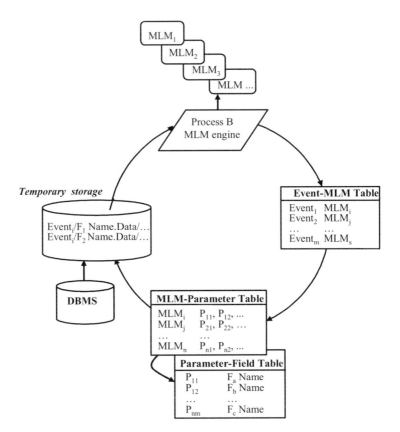

Figure 7.16: System mechanism with temporary storage.

Summary and Conclusions

Knowledge is difficult to define and is a messy and complex concept. Although we understand the difference between data, information, and knowledge the definitions become blurry. Knowledge is everywhere in the organization.

Knowledge-based systems (KBSs) will play an increasing role in the coming decades. Although early KBSs were built on rule-based formalisms that were mainstream in the 1980s, the strengths and weaknesses of this technology have been recognized and there has been an evolution to more comprehensive problem-solving methods. Reusable software components facilitate the implementation and maintenance of KBSs.

Today, KBSs must operate within clinical information systems (CISs) and community health information networks (CHINs) across a possibly heterogeneous computing environment. They must be integrated with clinical practice; hence they have evolved toward application spheres that support therapeutic-oriented activities instead of observation-oriented activities.

Guideline implementation is a key issue, and several standards have been proposed to model them with the underlying information system. Semantic intregration that should facilitate the mapping of concepts between record- and knowledge-based system remains a key research issue.

References

[Barahona 1994a] Barahona P, Christensen JP. Knowledge processing for decision support in the health sector. A perspective for the next decade. In: Baranona P, Christensen J (eds). *Knowledge and Decisions in Health Telematics*. Amsterdam: IOS Press, 1994.

[Barahona 1994b] Barahona P. The EPISTOL study part 1—the scenario report. In: Baranona P, Christensen J (eds). *Knowledge and Decisions in Health Telematics*. Amsterdam: IOS Press, 1994; pp. 3–58.

[Buchanan 1984] Buchanan GB, Shortliffe EH. *Rule-based Expert Systems. The MYCIN Experiments of the Stanford Heuristic Programming Project.* Reading: Addison-Wesley, 1984.

[Cannon 1980] Cannon ST, Gardner RM. Experience with a computerized interactive protocol system using HELP. *Comp Biomed Res.* 1980; 13: 399–409.

[Chute 1999] Chute CG, Elkin PL, Sherertz DD, Tuttle MS. Desiderata for a clinical terminology server. *JAMIA.* 1999; 6(suppl): 42–46.

[Cimino 1989] Cimino JJ, Hripcsak G, Johnson SB, Clayton PD. Designing an introspective, controlled medical vocabulary. In: Kingsland LW (ed). *Proc 13th Annual Symp on Computer Applications in Medical Care.* Washington, DC: IEEE Computer Society Press, 1989; pp. 513–580.

[Cimino 1994] Cimino JJ, Clayton PD, Hripcsak G, Johnson SB. Knowledge-based approaches to the maintenance of a large controlled medical terminology. *JAMIA.* 1994; 1(1): 35–50.

[Cimino 2001] Cimino JJ. Terminology tools: state of the art and practical lessons. *Meth Inform Med.* 2001; 40(4): 298–306.

[Davis 1993] Davis R, Shrobe H, Szolovits P. What is a knowledge representation? *AI Magazine.* 1993; 14(1): 17–33.

[Degoulet 1995] Degoulet P, Fieschi M, Chatellier G. Decision support systems from the standpoint of knowledge representation. *Methods Inform Med.* 1995; 34: 202–208.

[Elkin 2000] Elkin PL, Peleg M, Lacson R, Bernstam E, Tu S, Boxwala A, Greenes R, Shortliffe EH. Toward the standardization of electronic guidelines. *MD Comp.* 2000; 17(6): 39–44.

[Field 1990] Field M, Lohr K. Guidelines for clinical practice:Directions for a new program. Washington, DC: Institute of Medicine, National Academy Press; 1990.

[Fox 1998] Fox J, Thomson R. Decision support and disease management: a logic engineering approach. *IEEE Transact Inform Techno Biomed.* 1998; 2(4): 1–12.

[Genesereth 1994] Genesereth MR, Fikes RE. Knowledge Interchange Format. Version 3.0. Reference Manual. Stanford, CA: Stanford University, 1994. [http://logic.stanford.edu/kif/Hypertext/kif-manual.html].

[Glaser 2002] Glaser J. Experiences with knowledge applications in Medical Care. *J Health Care Information Management.* 2002;16 (2): 23–34.

[Gordon 1999] Gordon C, Veloso M. Guidelines in healthcare: the experience of the Prestige project. *Stud Health Technol Inform.* 2000;77: 23–28.

[Grimson 1988] Grimson J. Knowledge-base approach to hospital information systems. In: Bakker et al. (eds). *Towards New Hospital Information Systems.* North-Holland, Amsterdam: Elsevier, 1988; pp. 265–271.

[Haas 1986] Haas IL. The integration of data and knowledge base systems: activities in ESPRIT. Entity-relationship approach: ten years of experience in information modelling. *Proc 5th Inter Conf.* 1986; 9–21.

[Hayes-Roth 1994] Hayes-Roth F, Jacobstein N. The state of knowledge based systems. *Commun ACM.* 1994; 37(3): 27–39.

[Haynes 1990] Haynes RB, McKibbon KA, Walker CJ. Online access to MEDLINE in clinical setting. A study of use and usefulness. *Ann Intern Med.* 1990; 112(1): 78–94.

[Healthfield 1994] Heathfield HA, Wyatt J. Philosophies for the design and development of clinical decision-support systems. In: Van Bemmel J, McCray A (eds). Stuttgart: Schattauer, *Yearbook of Medical Informatics,* 1994; p. 332 –339.

[Hongying 1995] Hongying M. Medical logic modules based on the Arden syntax and hospital information systems. *Med Inform,* 1995; 20(1): 83–93.

[Lanzola 1993] Lanzola G, Stefanelli M. A specialized framework for medical diagnostic knowledge-based systems. *Comput Biomed Res.* 1992; 25(4): 351–365.

[Lincoln 1991] Lincoln MJ, Turner CW, Haug PJ, Warner HR, Williamson JW, Bouhaddou O, Jessen SG, Sorensen D, Cundick RC, Grant M. Iliad training enhances medical students' diagnostic skills. *J Med Syst.* 1991; 15(1): 93–110.

[Miller 1982] Miller RA, Pople ME, Myers JD. Internist-1, an experimental computer-based diagnostic consultant for general internal medicine. *N Engl J Med.* 1982; 307(8): 468–476.

[Miller 1986] Miller P. *Expert Critiquing Systems: Practice-Based Medical Consultation by Computer.* New York: Springer-Verlag, 1986.

[Miller 1990] Miller RA, Mararie FE. The demise of the "Greek oracle" model for medical diagnostic systems. *Methods Inform in Med.* 1990; 29(1): 1–2.

[Miller 1994] Miller RA. Taking inventory of medical decision support software development. In: Van Bemmel J, McCray A (eds). *Yearbook of Medical Informatics. Advanced Communication in Health Care, IMIA.* Stuttgart: Schattauer,1994; pp. 340–342.

[Minsky 1975] Minsky M. A framework for representing knowledge. In: Winston P (ed). *The Psychology of Computer Vision.* New York: McGrawHill, 1975; pp. 211–277.

[Musen 1993] Musen MA. Dimensions of knowledge sharing and reuse. In: In: Van Bemmel J, McCray A (eds). Stuttgart: Schattauer, *Yearbook of Medical Informatics. Sharing Knowledge and Information,* 1993; p. 402–421.

[Musen 1996] Musen M, Tu S, Das A, Shahar Y. EON: a component-based approach to automation of protocol-directed therapy. *JAMIA.* 1996; 3(6): 367–388.

[Negnevitsky 2001] Negnevitsky M. *Artificial Intelligence. A Guide to Intelligence Systems.* Harlow, Essex: Addison-Wesley, 2001.

[Ohno-Machado 1998] Ohno-Machado L, Gennari JH, Murphy S, Jain NL, Tu SW, Oliver DE, Pattison-Gordon E, Greenes RA, Shortliffe EH, Barnett GO. The guideline interchange format: a model for representing guidelines. *JAMIA.* 1998; 5(4): 357–372.

[OMG 1997] OMG. *Lexicon Query Services.* [http://www.omg.org/docs/corbamed/97-01-02.htm].

[Peleg 2000] Peleg M, Boxwala AA, Ogunyemi O, Zeng Q, Tu S, Lacson R, Bernstam E, Ash N, Mork P, Ohno-Machado L, Shortliffe EH, Greenes RA. GLIF3: the evolution of a guideline representation format. *Proc AMIA Symp.* 2000; pp. 645–649.

[Pryor 1993] Pryor TA, Hripcsak G. Sharing MLM's: an experiment between Columbia-Presbyterian and LDS Hospital. *Proc Annu Symp Comput Appl Med Care.* 1993; pp. 399–403.

[Rector 1995] Rector AL, Solomon WD, Nowlan WA, et al. A terminology server for medical language and medical information systems. *Methods Inform Med.* 1995; 34(1–2): 147–157.

[Rector 2001] Clinical terminology: why is it so hard? In: *Yearbook of Medical Informatics.* In: Van Bemmel J, McCray A (eds). Stuttgart: Schattauer, 2001; pp. 286–299.

[Rennels 1987] Rennels DG, Shortliffe HE. Advanced computing for medicine. *Sci Am.* 1987; Oct; 257(4); 154–161.

[Rocha 1994] Rocha RA, Huff SM, Haug PJ, Warner HR. Designing a controlled medical vocabulary server: the VOSER project. *Comp Biomed Res.* 1994; 27(6): 472–507.

[Shiffman 2000] Shiffman R, Nath S. *A preliminary evaluation of guideline content mark-up using GEM—an XML.* Guideline elements model. *Proc AMIA Annu Symp.* 2000; pp. 413–417.

[Shortliffe 1976] Shortliffe EH. *Computer-Based Medical Consultation: MYCIN.* New York: American Elsevier, 1976.

[Shortliffe 1993] Shortliffe EH. The adolescence of AI in medicine: will the field come of age in the '90s? *AI Med.* 1993; 5: 93–106.

[Sittig 1994] Sittig DF. Grand challenges in medical informatics. *JAMIA.* 1994; 1: 412–413.

[Sugden 1999] Sugden B, Purves IN, Booth N, Sowerby M. The PRODIGY project —the interactive development of the release one model. *AMIA Symp.* 1999; 359–363.

[Talmon 1990] Talmon JL. Knowledge-based systems, concepts, methods and techniques. In: Pretschner DR, Urrutia B (eds). *Knowledge-Based Systems to Aid Medical Image Analysis.* Commission of the E.C., DC Science, Research and Development,1990; pp. 11–12.

[Teach 1981] Teach RL, Shortliffe EH. An analysis of physician attitudes regarding computer-based clinical consultation systems. *Comput Biomed Res.* 1981; 14(6): 542–558.

[Tu 2000] Tu SW, Musen MA. Representation formalisms and computational methods for modeling guideline-based patient care. *First European Workshop on Computer-based Support for Clinical Guidelines and Protocols,* Leipzig, Germany, 2000; pp. 125–142.

[Tusch 1990] Tusch GM, Reichertz PL. Tools and shells for knowledge-based systems in medicine. In: Pretschner DP, Urrutia. B (eds). *Knowledge-Based Systems to Aid Medical Image Analysis.* Commission of the European Communities. EUR Report 12796, 1990; pp. 41–62.

[Van der Lei 1994] Van der Lei J. Computer-based decision support: the unfulfilled promise. In: Barahona P, Christensen JP (eds.) *Knowledge and Decisions. Health Telematics.* Amsterdam: IOS Press, 1994; pp. 67–72.

[Vissers 1995] Vissers MC, Hasman A, van der Linden CJ. Consultation behaviour of residents supported with a protocol processing system (Proto VIEW) at the emergency ward. *Int J Biomed Comp.*1995; 38: 181–187.

[Winston 1984] Winston PH. *Artificial Intelligence,* 2nd ed. Reading, MA: Addison-Wesley, 1984.

[Winston 1992] Winston PH. *Artificial Intelligence,* 3rd ed. Reading, MA: Addison-Wesley, 1992.

8

The Resource Management Component

Resource management is one of the key objectives of any healthcare organization. Resources include personnel (e.g., physicians, nurses, secretaries), space (e.g., consulting rooms, operating rooms), as well as the materials or consumables needed during a medical procedure. Resource management applications can maximize the efficiency of healthcare delivery. They can improve resource use, achieve more efficient care, and provide a high return on investment.

For the most part, resource allocation in hospitals is still done manually due to the fact that patients' appointments are managed by departmental applications that do not recognize the multiple interactions between complex medical procedures. Such a situation can lead to patient dissatisfaction (e.g., excessive waiting times), physician dissatisfaction (e.g., too much time wasted on scheduling activities because of unanswered phone calls or busy signals), and an overall loss of revenue for the institution (e.g., under-used equipment).

This chapter provides a broad overview of the essential building blocks and requirements for a resource management component. It focuses on the development and implementation of an enterprise-wide patient scheduling system. Most of the existing systems include scheduling functions but they do not meet all the requirements of a hospital-wide scheduling system. Furthermore, hospital-wide scheduling systems offer more features than do schedulers that are part of a departmental (or stand-alone) system.

Although there is considerable interest in optimizing patient appointment scheduling over a long period [Holston 1967, Peterson 1984, Vissers 1978, Zwieten-Edelenbos 1981] few (user-friendly) systems have been successfully installed. Patients (i.e., the demand side) and physicians (i.e., the supply side) have different viewpoints. As physicians deal with many patients but generally with one at a time, the personal efficiency of healthcare providers in general must be increased, providing better communications between professionals and better feedback. On the other hand, patients often view physicians and the hospital as a single entity. Efficient scheduling is a necessary step to guarantee the continuity of care.

Conceptual Specifications

Nature and Types of Resources

A resource can best be described as that which healthcare organizations consume or use in meeting their goals. A resource may be *passive* (or *consumable*) such as disposables, food, medications, and so on, or *active* (or *temporal),* such as medical equipment, facilities, rooms, buildings, and so on, to be used over time (Figure 8.1). A temporal resource can be described by its time availability (time slots). Resources also include people, information, and cash flow. Objects that are considered agents may also be considered resources.

Resource management includes acquisition (equipment, personnel), scheduling (patient appointment, nurse rosters), maintenance of devices, and disposal.

Resource classes	Subclasses
Healthcare staff	Physicians, nurses, pharmacists, administrative personnel
Organizational units	Ward units Ancillary services
Materials	Generic consumables Sterilized objects (to be identified individually) Drugs
Equipment	Clinical equipment Nonclinical equipment

Figure 8.1: Classification of resources in a healthcare organization.

Figure 8.1 summarizes the main classes of resources to be considered for the development of a generic resource management component. According to the capacities of the resource, three subcategories can be defined: global, unary and composite resources (Figure 8.2). In a medical environment, unary resources and composite resources (or pool resources) are the focus of patient scheduling systems.

Scheduling Systems

Scheduling is a constraint-based decision-making process in which resource-demanding activities are assigned to resources over time and comply with predefined constraints (Figure 8.3).

An *activity* requires, consumes, or produces a resource. Resolving a scheduling problem means dedicating one or more time slots to a specific requested item type (e.g., activity, medication, delivery) corresponding to a requested way or type of provisioning or ordering (externally, internally).

Resource type	Definition
Global	A resource whose capacity may vary over time (i.e., time units). Has a *minimum* and *maximum* capacity at each time unit. Required (provided) by activities in the schedule.
Unary	A resource whose maximum capacity is always one. Allows implementation of disjunctive constraints (i.e., some activities cannot occur simultaneously). For example, every medical device is a unary resource.
Composite	Represents a resource pool of undifferentiated resources whose capacity is defined by the amount of resources available over a given period of time rather than at each time unit. Has a minimum and maximum capacity over a time period (e.g., from 9 to 12 A.M.).

Figure 8.2: Categorization of scheduling resource classes.

When scheduling a particular appointment, the resource component needs to take into account the organizational constraints (e.g., certain scheduling desks can accommodate only certain types of medical activities), the medical constraints (e.g., certain activities to be scheduled need to be controlled against the medical history of the patient), and patient preferences (e.g., patients prefer specific physicians, are not always available). The scheduling engine performs optimization to determine the solution that best meets the conflicting preferences of each actor (patient, healthcare professional, administrator).

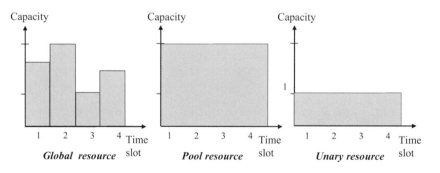

Figure 8.3: Resource capacity evolution.

Other constraints that affect the scheduling process in medicine include the activity duration, the pre- and postconditions of the activity, resource availability, the degree of urgency, and the inventory levels of required consumables.

Figure 8.4 presents an object-oriented model of the different resource classes to be managed by a resource component. Resource allocation is a task in which the complexity of the problem grows exponentially as more parameters and constraints are considered [Berger 1993].

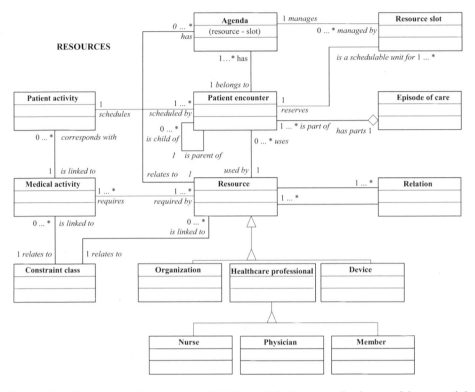

Figure 8.4: Scheduling object-oriented (OO) model. Conceptual schema of the essential classes managed by the resource component.

Functional Specifications

In most situations, an appointment is the step (task) that immediately follows the process of ordering an activity by a healthcare professional. In this context, patient appointment and scheduling systems offer the foundation upon which the order entry and result reporting subsystem, the medical record, and nursing IS may be built. This comprehensive view aims to bring the patient, the physician, and the medical record together at an appointed time. Within this framework, it is interesting to consider the objectives of a scheduling system for each category of participant.

Objectives of a Scheduling System

Patient's Point of View

From the patient's point of view, the objectives of a scheduling system are
- to reduce waiting times, and
- to achieve more individually oriented care and improve continuity of treatments (e.g., through a better flow of procedures).

Figure 8.5 summarizes the benefits of an automated scheduling system as compared to a traditional manual one.

Manual patient scheduling systems	Automated distributed scheduling systems
Appointments can be made only in dedicated units.	Appointments can be made from any terminal. By accessing the scheduling system, users at each location can view clinical department schedules any time and are able to make appointments at a time convenient for the patient.
For different services, different secretaries must be contacted.	The patient need to contact only one secretary.
Appointments are made only during working hours.	Appointments are made at any time.
When a patient forgets his appointment date, it becomes difficult to retrace the information.	Appointment schedules of patients are always available.
Cancellation of an appointment involves a lot of search and clerical work.	Canceling an appointment automatically generates messages to all the professionals involved.
For several appointments per patient, intensive telephone traffic is required.	Telephone traffic is reduced.
Statistical information available only with intensive efforts.	Statistical information can easily be inferred from the recorded data.
Many mistakes are made in identifying patients.	Patient identification mistakes are reduced.
Appointment reminders have to be sent out manually.	Reminders are automatically printed and/or e-mailed. This is especially useful for procedures that are scheduled on a recurring basis.
Communication with central medical archives is done only with a copying system.	Communication is automatically established.

Figure 8.5: Manual versus automatic scheduling systems.

Health Professional's Point of View

Physicians and nurses are concerned with the multiplicity and diversity of medical activities that can benefit from scheduling systems. Searching for the best available time slots based on patient preferences and resource availability with a scheduling system reduces the time needed to search through multiple schedule charts for an optimum combination of appointments. Objectives for healthcare professionals include the following:

- minimizing the delay between the request for a medical activity and its execution;
- being informed of the status of scheduled activities; and
- reducing the time spent in the appointment management process (e.g., phone calls).

Administrator's Point of View

Administrators have the following objectives:
- to improve communications between the various departments;
- to reduce the time spent in collecting, processing, and supplying information;
- to reduce the number of professionals involved in the administration of appointments;
- to spread out patient appointments over the full workday and reduce peak periods; and
- to improve professional efficiency and resource utilization (personnel, materials).

Various customized reports (mostly unavailable in manual systems) can contribute information to achieve these goals. They include resource utilization statistics (e.g., underuse or inadequate use of equipment, time and space occupancy), lists of no-shows, and canceled appointments (e.g., uncooperative patients) (Figure 8.6).

Requirements of a Scheduling System

The requirements of a patient scheduling system can be categorized at the patient, service planning, activity scheduling, management, and integration levels.

Patient Level

- Patients should be easily identified easily, so that appointments can be made by phone or e-mail. The following ways of accessing the central database should be available: soundex (phonetic), family name, date of

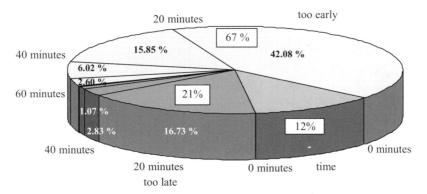

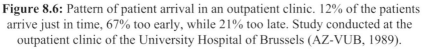

Figure 8.6: Pattern of patient arrival in an outpatient clinic. 12% of the patients arrive just in time, 67% too early, while 21% too late. Study conducted at the outpatient clinic of the University Hospital of Brussels (AZ-VUB, 1989).

birth, and patient ID number. To speed up the scheduling process, "smart" cards, magnetic cards that identify the patient can be used (see Chapter 6).

- It should not be necessary to first identify the patient before booking an appointment. The scheduler first looks for a free slot, verifies if it suits the patient, and if so, then identifies the patient and displays the open appointments and/or past appointments.

- Scheduling can be carried out on an individual basis or for a group of patients (students, employees on behalf of employer, etc.).

- Facilities are requested to trace patients from their arrival to their departure.

- Transportation requests for inpatients are generated based on their mobility.

- If more than one examination is planned, the system should assist in choosing the best possible schedule.

- The scheduling system should

  - provide the full schedule of a patient within the entire system;

  - schedule appointments for known (registered: inpatient and outpatient) and unknown (not registered) patients, as well as resources, facilities, and medical equipment;

  - schedule multiple appointments (for different clinical departments) for the same patient (with reduced stay time or fewer outpatient walkins);

  - schedule during one transaction, a number of patients, for the same appointment (i.e. the same medical procedure, same clinical department);

  - link multiple fixed and consumable resources used for the appointment; and

- reschedule and transfer appointments, and inform patients through cancellation notices. Rescheduling functions include block schedule moves and cancellations.

- If an appointment is made for a patient (as inpatient or outpatient), it should be possible to change the patient's status (e.g., change inpatient status into outpatient status).

- Extra attention should be paid to patients who must be seen as quickly as possible because of high medical priority (e.g., patients sent by the emergency unit, or inpatients). For some medical services it is therefore advisable to keep some slots open at regular intervals.

- New patients and special patients (e.g., V.I.P., infected) can be registered and no-show patients can be noted.

Service-Planning Level

- It should be possible to draw up individual templates (appointment diaries) in a user-friendly way for every clinical (or administrative) resource unit.

  - Scheduling is calendar-based on predefined time slot parameters and templates.

  - The scheduling grid allows both block time (several patients per time slot) or open time (one patient per time slot) in variable time increments.

  - Each template may further be subdivided into specific scheduling programs. For example, a physician can choose to see two patients for 30 minutes each in the first hour of the day, then see eight patients for 15 minutes each in the second and third hour, and then see three patients for 20 minutes each in the fourth hour.

  - Scheduling exceptions, such as weekends, and maintenance, can be accommodated.

- Some scheduling algorithms consider the availability of only one resource, whereas others also consider the availability of multiple resources, such as technicians and machines. This is defined as the multiple resource booking facility.

- The resource administrator is designed to accommodate clinical departments' policies. Depending on the circumstances, the planning and authorization profile can be adjusted. Thus, it should be possible to do the following:

  - Block (and transfer) an appointment unit in advance for a certain period for a specific reason (maintenance, holiday, etc.).

  - Allow the resource administrator to define other user authorization profiles (privileges). Booking certain procedures can be reserved for specific user groups.

- Allow overruling facilities by user, type of resource, and medical procedure. For example, in the radiology department two successive radiologic procedures will take less time than doing the two procedures individually.

- Allow automatic conflict checking: drawing attention to the incompatibility between certain examinations, for example, intravenous pyelography after an examination of the stomach or CT scan after an examination of the stomach with contrast. Other features generate relevant questions: Is the patient pregnant? Does a patient scheduled for an MRI have metal prostheses?

- Define access by department or user profile. For example, if the cardiology department needs at least 20 minutes for an ECG, the centralized scheduler won't allow more than one patient to be scheduled in any 20-minute period.

- Specify overbooking, which can lead to excessive pressure on physicians and technicians who have to see more patients in the same time interval (time slot). Therefore, a tool is needed to control and assess the degree of overbooking.

- Keep appointment slots free for emergencies.

• The computerized scheduling system needs built-in logic (rules):

- checks for medical and organizational conflicts, and

- controls who is allowed to schedule resources or to use the DISPLAY, PLAN, REGISTER, and DELETE PERMISSIONS options.

• A centralized and a decentralized scheduling feature must be available:

- centralized multipurpose scheduling provides access across multiple medical departments from one location,

- decentralized single purpose scheduling provides access for only one medical department from different locations, and

- decentralized multipurpose scheduling provides access across multiple medical departments from several (functional) locations.

• A computerized patient scheduling system can operate in a manual or an automatic mode. In the manual mode, the secretary highlights the patient and enters examinations, preferred time, and physician (or room), according to the type of examination and priorities. When an automatic mode is selected, the system will present the first available time slot for the first physician (or examination room) available, based on predefined criteria. Here, rooms, physicians, and examinations are defined with the interrelations between them.

• Features must also be available to schedule resources (e.g., meeting rooms) for nonpatient purposes, such as staff meetings.

Activity Level

- The scheduler makes selections from a list of predefined procedures, each procedure with its own constraints (precedence, duration, etc.).

- Scheduling instructions or activity instructions are provided for the user. Every time an appointment is assigned, the scheduled event (date, time, place) with all additional information (e.g., special instructions for the clinical procedure) should be displayed or printed out on an appointment sheet for the patient. For example, a patient should be told not to eat or drink after a certain time the day before an appointment for a particular test or medical procedure.

- Booking of protocols or "batteries" of medical activities can be done in a time sequence with additional medical and/or organizational constraints.

- Sometimes there is a need to reschedule. For some medical areas (radiotherapy, chemotherapy, etc.) rescheduling is an important feature that necessitates *a schedule revision* algorithm as opposed to a *schedule construction* algorithm. The schedule revision algorithms' response time must be a few seconds. For example, if a clinical department changes its hours of operation for a particular medical test, the scheduling office can quickly update its schedule roster. Or if a physician is ill, his appointments will be canceled and patients will be informed.

- Users who interact with the patient appointment and scheduling system must be provided with a reliable graphical user interface (GUI) that gives them access to the system via customized displays resembling their usual agenda as much as possible (e.g., scheduled cases are represented by different colors for available, booked, overbooked, canceled appointments). It displays current and future allocations in a comprehensively designed graphical layout format. The colors and symbols must be designed to be very intuitive to end-users and must present overviews:

  - *By patient:* requested, scheduled, rejected, no-show.

  - *By resource:* orthogonal occupational views:
    - one resource (or multiple resources) versus time periods;
    - patients versus time periods by resource (work list), by referring department.
    - global views (average) occupancy over a specific period by resource or by appointment type.

  - *By activity:* activities on an individual or group level can be represented with a user-defined color.

- When necessary, the scheduling module creates supply requisitions that are used for billing and inventory purposes, prints appointment reminder notices for patients, prints transportation lists, and provides information on completed appointments, no shows, late arrivals, walk-in patients, and emergency visits (optionally through bar coding).

Management Level

A scheduling system assists the hospital in managing outpatient and inpatient visits and provides managers with better control of the human and other resources they need to manage.

The system provides control information about the visiting patterns, and occupancy profiles at the departmental and enterprise level of the hospital. The previous illustration of a waiting-time situation (Figure 8.6) is based on the registered data of 12,000 patients from the University Hospital in Brussels (700 beds, 300,000 polyclinic visits per year, 1988). Figure 8.7 shows that, on the average, patients

- enter the hospital 15 minutes earlier than necessary;

- are present 6 minutes before the time set up for the doctor's consultation; and

- have to wait 24 minutes after the time set up for the consultation, which takes up about 10 minutes.

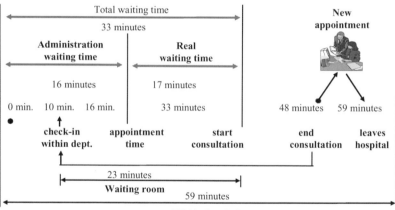

Figure 8.7: Waiting-time situation. Study conducted in the Orthopedic Clinic, University Hospital of Brussels (AZ -VUB 1989).

For a certain period of time the following information should be made available:

• planned and actual visits (inpatients versus outpatients);

• unplanned, no-shows, and emergency visits;

• first and subsequent visits (what was the percentage of new patients seen in each clinic?);

• activity profile statistics: average occupancy;

• planned and actual opening hours (how long did it take to see the physician?);

• sum totals per physician, specialty, working day, period, apparatus;

- percentage of occupancy (what is the waiting time?);
- trends per numbers of patients per specialty; and
- referrals via outside physicians (general practitioners, specialists) and referral ratio.

Integration Level

A scheduling system is not a stand-alone application. The system must be seamlessly integrated with existing HISs, POEs, and EHRs providing a bi-directional flow of data in order to be consistent. The interface engine supports both incoming (requests for activities to be scheduled from POE patient updates, e.g., changing inpatient locations, and other modifications) and outgoing (scheduling results, activity status, etc.) data streams.

The resource scheduling component is integrated with the following components:

- *The patient component*

    - for known patients from the patient identification (PID) server to the resource scheduling server; and

    - for unknown patients from the resource scheduling server to the PID server concerning information gathered during the scheduling process.

- *The activity component*

    - Orders generated by the activity component must be sent via e-mail and scheduled (manually or automatically).

    - The scheduling result must be transmitted on-line to the appropriate requester. Information in the scheduling system will be the basis for the nursing care plan.

Formats to exchange data can be HL7, XML, etc., compliant. It is clear that one of the fundamental components of this scheduling application is the workflow system.

Scheduling Templates

When a scheduling system is introduced, one of the most important tasks is to define an appointment schedule or template indicating how many patients can be expected to be treated in a certain period of time (Figure 8.8). The definition or specification of all the accompanying scheduling prerequisites for the scheduling system leads to the design of a "template" similar to a page in an appointment diary. The great difference between systems for appointment administration lies in the refinement of these templates:

- How many templates can be created per doctor or group of doctors?

- A scheduling calendar that is based on predefined time parameters, slot lengths, and templates (diagrams), can accommodate
  - variable-length appointments, and
  - fixed-length appointments defining the number of patients allowed per time slot.

- Overbooking facilities for specific resources at certain time slots/intervals.

- Protocols including a predefined sequence of activities across multiple services related to pathology, surgery and so on.

• Are multiple schemes proposed (by day, by department, etc.)?

• Are time data (day of the week, days of leave, etc.) taken into account when templates are being drawn up?

• Is it possible to introduce flexible consulting hours?

• Is it possible to reserve parts of appointments periodically (for instance, for the maintenance of equipment)?

• What time frame can be covered? Some systems are limited to a maximum of 3 months, whereas some medical departments need a 1- to 2-year appointment time frame. Sometimes it is also advisable, from the point of view of patient service, to register for later processing the actual time and length of the consultation for each patient.

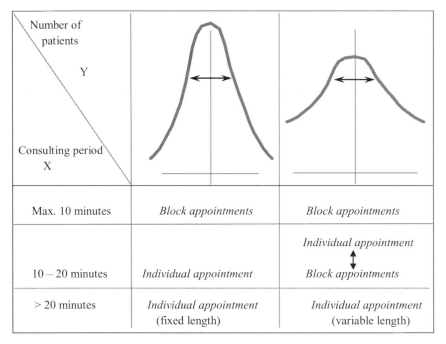

Max. 10 minutes	*Block appointments*	*Block appointments*
10 – 20 minutes	*Individual appointment*	*Individual appointment* ↕ *Block appointments*
> 20 minutes	*Individual appointment* (fixed length)	*Individual appointment* (variable length)

Figure 8.8: Outline schedule of possible appointment systems in relation to the deviation; X, length of examination; Y, number of patients.

Choosing the Optimum Appointment Schedule

The selected appointment schedule depends on two factors: the average length and the deviation length of an examination (treatment) (Figure 8.8) [Schuling 1973]. For examinations of very short duration the pure block (group) schedule is better (Figure 8.9).

Two-at-a-time: several patients at each appointment time
At one appointment time, two (or several) patients are scheduled. This system is advised for doctors who limit themselves to short consulting times, thus generating a a higher occupation percentage.
Individual system: fixed duration of examination
With the individual appointment schedule, one appointment per unit of time is made. The individual appointment per hour is recommended for longer consultations, in the event of a large difference between consultation intervals (from 15 minutes to an hour). The system reduces the waiting time for patients and allows them to arrive closer to the time they will be seen.
Block appointments (pure block system): several patients at the same time
This system schedules all patients at the same time—when the clinic opens. Patients are taken care of on a first-come, first-served basis. The patient is not given an appointment for a specific hour, but all the patients are told to come at the same time. The advantage for the physicians is that they will always have patients, and in case a patient does not arrive or comes too late, the physician continues working and will not be kept waiting for the patients. On the other hand, the advantages for the patients are less obvious because they have to wait their turn. This type of block appointment system will work fine if the number of patients to be seen is relatively small or if the average time that a physician spends with each patient is short.
Walk-in patients: completely free consulting hours
This system is often found with general practitioners. The patient comes during consulting hours. Again, the rule is first-come, first-served.
Variable length: Individual appointment schedule with a variable length of consultation
This is comparable to the individual appointment schedule, but the length of each consultation depends on the patient and on the medical treatment. It is recommended for medical services or physicians who need a rather long and varying time interval, which depends on each patient, treatment, or medical activity (e.g., psychiatrists).

Figure 8.9: Depending on the consulting physician's work method, or the department in question, several types of appointment schedules can be used [Van de Velde 1992].

For consultations of longer duration, the individual appointment schedule is preferred. Furthermore, the general conclusion that can be drawn is that the more personal the appointment (with a particular doctor at a specified time), the lower the "no-show" rate of patients and the better the punctuality of both doctors and patients. The ultimate aim is one appointment per unit of time because this causes the waiting time of the patients to be reduced to a minimum.

Activity	Express (time and other) constraints of and between activities
Temporal	• Preparation time of an activity • Precedence relationship (sequence, time) - start after: end of activity + Δt; start of activity + Δt - end after: end of activity + Δt; start of activity + Δt • Activity duration dependent on some variables (e.g., patient type, inpatient, outpatient) • Conflict checking (e.g., scheduled activities at the same time)
Number	• Combinatorial rules of activities - Compulsory, e.g., if activity A, then always with B (or + C + x) - Prohibited, e.g., A and B not allowed • Maximum/minimum number of activities allowed • Same activity previously been scheduled "x time" ago • Activity guidelines
Resource availability	**Express conditions under which a resource may be used**
	• Human resource availability: vacation, unavailability, etc. • Passive resource: maintenance, availability of other resources • The concurrent availability of several resources • The availability of other resources: active and passive, e.g., equipment, medication, and disposable
Resource utilization	**Express how activities make use of resources**
	• Require a resource temporarily: patient consultation • Consume a resource permanently: medication administering, consumables, etc. • Provide a resource temporarily • Produce a resource permanently
Patient constraints	**Express constraints from medical or patient point of view**
	• Diagnosis-related, e.g., if diagnosis = X, then activity A • Patient age-related • Patient sex-related • Patient type-related (e.g., new patient, first-time visit, inpatient, outpatient) • Preference(s) from patient (time, resource), group of patients

Figure 8.10: Scheduling constraints.

Subsequently, it should be checked regularly whether an adjustment of the chosen schedule is necessary. This can be done, for instance, by roughly measuring the waiting times once a year. Constraints can be checked concurrently (Figure 8.10).

Parameters to Be Considered

A number of parameters must be determined before assigning an appointment to a patient. It is also important to consider the patient's personal wishes. The following parameters are considered in scheduling an appointment:

- *The length of a consultation/treatment*
  The total average length of the specified examination/treatment in that department (i.e., the interval between the time a patient enters and the time the medical service is ready for the next patient) must be known in advance.

- *The appointment time*
  The required time for consultation (according to the attending doctor's advice and according to the patient's wishes) in the short-term or in the long-term must be given. It has been found that patients tend to keep recently made appointments better. Therefore, it is necessary with long-term appointments to send a reminder to the patient, citing the date, time, and department (location) (and any documents that should be brought).

- *Additional examinations/treatments*
  It should be known whether or not the patient has to undergo any additional examinations. Therefore, the patient's flows to and between medical departments should be organized in such a way that the outpatient's number of visits to the outpatient department can be minimized.

- *Appointments arranged in the morning*
  This group includes all procedures for which the patient has to have an empty stomach and all other procedures occurring in combination with an examination on an empty stomach. Obviously, it is advisable to make appointments for all these activities on the same morning.

- *Interval*
  In some cases an intervening period between various consultations is necessary, for instance blood tests or cardiology tests in nuclear medicine.

- *Personal patient preferences*
  Some patients always request the same physician; either this must be reported to the computer as a parameter again and again, or the system memorizes this information.

Architecture of the Resource Component

Four subcomponents are essential building blocks for an enterprise-wide scheduling system: the activity thesaurus, the workflow engine, the scheduling engine, and the interface engine.

Activity Thesaurus

Medical activities, medical devices, and additional items useful for the scheduling of an activity or a sequence of activities are centralized in an activity thesaurus. The purpose is twofold:

- to provide the scheduling engine with ready-to-use information and constraints to generate (combined with personal patient preferences) one or more scheduling proposals as part of a batch run; and
- to extract from the main thesaurus a customized view per medical domain of the corresponding activity and resource classes with their corresponding attributes (name, synonyms, and administrative and billing data).

Workflow Engine

Almost all medical processes involve a number of tasks and activities performed by different users at different times at various locations. For example, when a physician places an order for an ECG, the supervising physician approves the requisition (business rule), and a cardiology secretary schedules an appointment and determines which cardiologist will take care of the patient. Concurrently, corresponding requests are forwarded to the transportation service (in case the patient needs transportation), and the requesting ward unit and physician are notified of this examination. Upon completion of the medical procedure, results are sent to one (or more) physicians inside or outside the hospital. Functional integration requires the modeling of healthcare processes as part of a business model and is achievable through the application of workflow management techniques. Medical activities must be routed and directed through an underlying workflow engine (see Chapter 5).

Scheduling Engine

Based on the knowledge and information stored in the activity thesaurus, the scheduling engine assigns activities to resources for a patient over time by allocating one or several time slots for a specific date and time in the future. An activity executes without interruption from t_{start} to t_{end}, during Δt. An activity requires (provides) the same resources throughout its execution. The scheduling engine enables physicians and managers to monitor and predict future workload and provides facilities to

- check availability of free slots;
- hold slots for urgent elective patients;
- have slots dedicated for specific medical procedures, each with its own resource requirement profile; and
- provide a number of alternative scheduling functions, such as cancellations, modification, and so on.

Two kinds of decisions are generated in the scheduling engine: time placement decisions (At what time should each activity be scheduled?) and resource allocation decisions (Which resources should be scheduled?).

A variety of constraints affect scheduling: duration of a medical activity, precedence constraints, preparation time and resource availability, environmental constraints (e.g., availability of other resources, inventory levels).

Interface Engine

The interface engine enables the integration of the resource component with the patient, activity, and knowledge components. An example of an interfaced scheduling system is given in Figure 8.11.

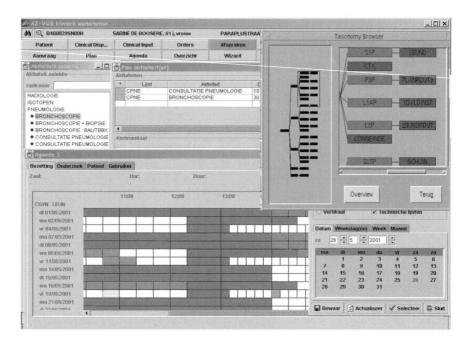

Figure 8.11: Resource management at the Brussels AZ-VUB University Hospital. Example of a scheduling and planning system as used by the radiotherapy department.

Summary and Conclusions

Solving resource allocation (people, medical devices, tasks, etc.) and scheduling problems in a heavily constrained environment is an essential and important task in many healthcare organizations in their attempt to operate in an ever more cost-efficient way. Reducing budgets will foster the importance of hospital-wide scheduling systems to provide better service to patients, improve resource utilization, and increase staff productivity.

State-of-the art scheduling systems should not be designed for a particular department but must be able to accommodate various medical systems and functions. This involves enterprise-wide as opposed to departmental thinking, or horizontal as opposed to vertical thinking.

The most important capabilities of comprehensive scheduling systems are centralized and decentralized scheduling features, block and multiple resource scheduling (patient, provider, staff, rooms and equipment), incorporation of clinical and business rule-based scheduling, and adjustable resource pattern scheduling. Important management issues are overbooking, conflict checking, waiting list functions, cancellation tracking, no-shows rates and reschedules, and the availability of other audit trails. Integration with the other components remains crucial.

In introducing an automatic system for appointment administration, a number of very important questions have to be answered in advance:

- Who is going to assign the appointments (centralized versus decentralized)?
- Is overbooking allowed? If so, for which type of patients/examinations/treatments? Who is to decide on this?
- Are qualifying periods accommodated if, for specific reasons, an appointment cannot be assigned?
- How will the system deal with the cancellations of particular appointments?
- Who is going to draw up the appointment schedules per doctor/department?

There are disadvantages to automation as well:

- What is to be done in the case of a computer failure?
- How is the security problem solved?

The optimum solution depends on the on the size and organization of the institution (e.g., central versus scattered buildings). Additionally, the selection of an appointment administrator is a necessary condition for success.

References

[Berger 1993] Berger R. Constraint based gate allocation for airports. Singapore: Knowledge engineering. Pte Ltd, Changi International Airport Singapore. *Ilog Publication.* 1993. [http://www.ilog.com/products/optimization/tech/custpapers/soluc32.pdf].

[Holston 1967] Holston CA. Central appointment system for outpatient clinics. *Hosp Manag.* 1967; 65–71.

[Peterson 1984] Peterson GF. *PCS/ADS resource and appointments scheduling system.* IBM. International Customer Executive Program, 1984.

[Schuling 1973] Schuling J. *Het afspraak-spreekuur* (appointment hours). Doctorate Thesis. Groningen: Groningen University, 1973; 4.

[Van de Velde 1992] Van de Velde R. *Hospital Information Systems. The Next Generation.* Berlin: Springer-Verlag, 1992.

[Vissers 1978] Vissers JMH. Wachttijden in de polikliniek (Waiting times in the outpatient clinic). *Medisch Contact.* 1978; 500–503.

[Zwieten-Edelenbos 1981] Zwieten-Edelenbos HJ. Afspraakplanning als onderdeel van een totaal ziekenhuiscommunicatie- en informatiesysteem (Appointments scheduling as part of a complete hospital communication and data system). *Proc Medical Informatics Congress (MIC)* 1981, Medische Informatica–Informatique Medicale, Belgische Vereniging voor Medische Informatica (MIM-VMBI).

9

The Security Component

The confidentiality of information available to the providers and quality of care are strongly interrelated. Some security precautions mainly apply only to stored information (e.g., access rights), whereas others apply to communicated information (e.g., proof of origin) or to both categories (e.g., confidentiality). The guarantee that personal information will not be altered or tampered with is of great importance in keeping patients' confidence in the healthcare system. Patient information therefore must be handled in a secure and efficient way so that only authorized persons have access to it.

Medical information includes all information that the patient confides or that is collected in the therapeutic context, including information that is secondary generated and information that is not directly or indirectly linked to the provision of healthcare [CMA 1998].

A fundamental difference between information processing in the past and in the present is that users and resources, as part of a clinical information system, are situated both inside and outside the organization. Outside users may be as demanding as those inside. For instance, sharing electronic healthcare records among disparate organizations is a complex task that entails all the methods by which electronic healthcare records are made available to healthcare professionals. It includes accessing a physical healthcare record archive (database interrogation, access to record components), creating a virtual healthcare record by enabling access to data from several different sources (distributed database interrogation), and communicating healthcare records in whole or in part through messaging.

This chapter focuses on the security aspects that can be provided through a security component. The security component is responsible for, among other tasks, the management of the users' profiles based on the identity of users and the groups to which they belong. Those rules should define the tasks users may invoke, the data and other objects (such as files, directories, devices, and so on) they have access to, and the terms of access (e.g., read, write, or modify). The access policy should be based on the security policy defined by the security management committee of the institution and comply with the legal requirements.

Conceptual Specifications

Security Principles

Security

Security is a general term that covers all the precautions taken whenever health information is collected, used, disclosed, or accessed. Security is an attribute of any information system. Security includes the physical and technical tools required for assuring the availability, confidentiality, integrity, and accountability of information and critical services. Security protection can be broken down, according to the Department of Defense Trusted Computer Systems Evaluation Criteria (*The Orange Book*), into four broad hierarchical divisions of security protection levels (from D minimal to A1 maximal security) [DoD 1985].

Organizations need fine-grained access security to an adequate level of detail to control who can do what. In general, security measures can be categorized as access security, communication security, content security, and security management (Figure 9.1) [Titterington 2001].

Access security issues include user authorization management, user identification (including smart cards, biometric devices, and password/PIN-generating "key fobs"), firewalls, and digital certification and public key infrastructure (PKI) issues. *Access control* is the ability to limit and control the access to host systems and applications.

Communication security issues include security communications protocols that secure messages (encryption). Security protocols generally also provide authentication. The security protocols that have emerged on the Web are Netscape's SSL (Secure Sockets Layer), NCSA's SHTTP (Secure HTTP), PCT (Private Communications Technology) a protocol from Microsoft that provides secure transactions, and the IETF's IPSec (IP SECurity). Web browsers and servers generally support all the popular security protocols.

Content security issues include content filtering to eliminate undesirable content (from Web sites, files, databases, and communications), encrypted file storage and databases, and virus detection. Depending on the chosen data classification scheme the following protection goals are also included: data confidentiality, data integrity, and data availability.

Security management issues include security assessment, intrusion detection, vulnerabilities assessment, and support for the development and implementation of security policies and guidelines.

	Storage	Communication
Authentication and user identification	Validation of credentials Electronic signature	Digital signature Cryptography
Authorization and access control	Granting of rights Access control list	Not applicable
Confidentiality	Firewall	Encryption Secured networks: tunneling (VPN, SSL)
Availability	Replication Clustering Backup Redundancy	Virus scanning Redundancy (high availability)
Integrity	Input validation checking Virus scanning	Cryptography
Nonrepudiation	Not applicable	Digital signature
Auditing and monitoring	Failed login attempts Intrusion detection system alarms	Intrusion detection system

Figure 9.1: Security precautions applied to stored and communicated information. VPN—Virtual Private Network; SSL—Secure Socket Layer.

The major components of a security infrastructure that ensure an adequate level of protection and reliability for the overall system include [King 2001]: the *network* (firewalls, switches, routers that monitor and protect data traversing the network), the *physical components* (door keys, identification badges, biometric devices, etc.), the *platform* (encompasses server, client-software, and application-level access controls that include functions like authorization, authentication, intrusion detection, virus detection, etc.), and a *corporate security policy and procedural guidelines*.

Privacy

Privacy is the right of an individual to remain apart from other people and not be seen, heard, or disturbed by them. The protection concerns both physical and psychological intrusions, and the misuse and abuse of something legally owned by an individual or normally considered by society to be his or her property [EPIC 2002].

Confidentiality

Confidentiality is the obligation of the holder of identifiable personal information to protect the person's privacy. This obligation is determined by common practice, laws, and regulations, and may vary from country to country. Confidential information includes sensitive or secret information, and information for which unauthorized disclosure could be harmful or prejudicial [Iversen 1995].

In some situations, consent is explicitly given by patients (orally or in writing) to permit access to or collection, use or disclosure of their medical information for well-defined purposes. *Disclosure* means the provision of medical information from one professional to another.

Accountability

Accountability (traceability) is the possibility of clearly tracing back actions to certain individuals, that is to make them accountable. Accountability can be considered at the write/update level (a trace is kept for every change in a patient database) but also at the read level (user x has read part of record y at time t).

An *audit trail* is the common mechanism deployed to record and examine system activity. It ensures that all changes to business objects are recorded. Security logs are necessary on a daily basis to gather all logins used, all failed login attempts (e.g., TCP/IP addresses, login times, dates, and accessed pages), and all changes made to the databases.

Information Integrity

Information integrity is the preservation of content when accessing, updating, or copying data so that there is confidence that information is complete and has not been altered (accidentally or intentionally, e.g., during transmission other than authorized) [CMA 1998]. Integrity rules described during the modeling process of the databases can foster data integrity. They include static verification constraints (e.g., validation bounds) and dynamic constraints (e.g., delta checks for laboratory data).

Information and Resource Availability

Availability of medical information requires that precautions be undertaken to prevent loss or to recover certain resources of a system. Availability assures that authorized users have access to relevant information at the time and place and in the format needed. This implies that hardware and software failures causing downtime or loss of information (accidental or intentional) should be covered as much as possible by corresponding system management activities (e.g., redundant array of inexpensive disks RAID disks, backup procedures, clustered systems).

The achievement of defined objectives of throughput and latency is also important. In critical environments such as healthcare production systems, not meeting a predefined performance level is equivalent to a system failure.

Security Modeling

The clinical information system can be considered to be a set of components. From its internal perspective, each component interacts with various external agents that are either individual users or other components. Each component may be described in terms of a set of controlled functions whose invocation and manipulation by external agents is subject to specific authorizations, derived from the authorization profiles and a set of authorized classes of data [CEN 1999].

Rule	Description	Attributes
Healthcare actor	Identifies who is authorized to have access to patient data. Persons may be classified into groups.	Profession Specialization Healthcare organization Patient
Time frame	Temporal limits of the authorization procedure.	Valid from t_1 until t_2 Episode of care Episode description
Nodes	Defines where the authorized healthcare party (role) has access to information. A list of workstation(s) or node(s) of the overall information system from which the healthcare actor is allowed to interact with the object.	Organizational requirements
Criteria	Determines the criteria (purpose of use/role) that provide a healthcare professional (HCP) with rights to access data within the patient record.	Purpose of use by the healthcare professional Organizational requirements
Communication object type	How patient information will be made available or visualized.	Security policy Patient consent required Third-party consent Access type and method
Type of authorization	Functions provided by the system to be executed. Description of the security model.	Get patient record, modify encounter, etc. Data allowed for access (e.g., read, create, modify)

Figure 9.2: Examples of distribution rules.

Each authorization profile may operate with a set of controlled functions. This profile describes the criteria and rules according to which users may be authorized to access information and perform activities in their specific roles and responsibilities within the organization. The process of data distribution must be defined as a set of rules (Figure 9.2).

Each agent of the clinical information system is characterized by a name, a unique public identifier (e.g., a code), and some mechanisms (password, fingerprints, etc.) for ensuring correct identification. To access a component, the agent must be a member of the authorization profile of that component. Such membership is granted by another individual agent (the security administrator) and is valid for a specific time period (i.e., between a starting and an expiration date/time). For example a physician can generally work on a ward unit but be present from time to time in the emergency department.

Disclosure rules are required to decide to whom data can be provided and for which purpose, which specific actions a user may invoke against a file or through an application and for how long (period), under which conditions, and which procedures have to be followed to gain access to the information. An ongoing European pre–standard development project is currently studying a method for building a set of rules for sharing healthcare records [CEN 1999].

With respect to the standard authorizations specified for a user's profile, exceptions, in terms of extensions of, or limitations to, the authorizations of individual agents may be defined.

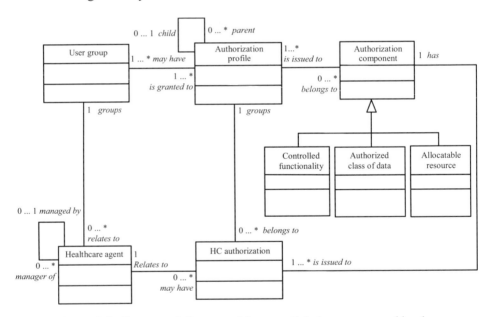

Figure 9.3: Conceptual diagram of the essential classes managed by the authorization module of a security component.

Figure 9.3 presents an object-oriented model of the different security classes to be managed by the authorization component. The authorization profile class contains all the authorization profiles defined in the information system and is related to a number of objects (authorization component) in terms of (subtypes) functionalities (controlled functionalities), data (authorized class of data), devices (allocatable resource), and so on. Agents belong to a specific class (user group) and can be an individual user, an organizational unit, a software component, and so on. The authorization profile of a specific agent is contained in the HC authorization object and may take on various values. A user may adopt different roles and the user/role relationship is time-limited.

Establishment of a Healthcare Security Policy

System requirements concern access, confidentiality, and the transfer of data. They must be supplemented by rules defined in a *security policy*. There is not a one-size-fits-all policy for all organizations, as well as most organizations cannot define a one-policy-fits-all approach. A healthcare security policy is a statement of the following [Cohen 1997]:

- The expectations of safety and confidentiality. It defines standards and guidelines as to how much and what kinds of security measures should be implemented.
- Procedures for the implementation of standards and guidelines to carry out the security policy—the rules (or laws) that the system must observe.
- The audits required to detect and record violations of the laws.

Security Issues When Accessing Health Data

Identification, Authentication, and Authorization

Confidentiality controls access to information and ensures that personal information is accessible only to authorized people. When logging onto a computer system, three security steps are generally considered:

1. *The identification step*: Who is the end-user?
2. *The authentication step*: Can the user prove it?
3. *The authorization step*: Is the user authorized to do what he/she intends to do?

Identification is the process of informing the system about the end-user's identity.

Authentication is the procedure used to verify that the user is the announced one. This proof of identity can follow three strategies:

1. Information shared by the system and the user (the user knows). This is the common situation in today's systems where the user provides identity elements such as the name, a personal identification number (PIN), and/or a password.
2. End-user's personal characteristics (that the user has). Every individual has a set of unique physiologic, behavioral, and morphologic characteristics that can be used for positive identification. Examples are retina

patterns, fingerprints, hand prints, voice pattern, key stroke, and signature patterns [Eberl 1997]. Such *biometric identification* has been in use for several years in highly secure areas such as military systems, but is now becoming more generalized.

3. A physical device (that the user holds). Examples of held devices are physical keys or cards (e.g., magnetic, optical, smart cards).

An example combining several approaches is the use of security hardware tokens, a small handheld device containing a microprocessor that calculates and displays random codes. These codes change at a specified interval, typically every 60 seconds. A session is initiated by entering a user name, a memorized PIN, and the currently displayed password from the secure device. This information is transmitted to a security server that authenticates the user and verifies that the correct password has been entered. The security server compares the user-entered password with its knowledge of which password should have been entered for that period. Once a password is verified, the user is authenticated for for the duration of the Web session. An encrypted security "cookie" is sent back to the user's browser and this cookie is automatically used for all future security dialogs. If a token is lost or stolen, it can be immediately deactivated for the entire activity by disabling it at the security server level.

Smart cards can be secured by adding biometric features. This greatly improves the security for the card holder in the event that the card is lost or stolen, and enables the confidence of the issuing organization that the individual it has allowed to access the computer network is the one who actually accesses it. Authentication is performed by comparing the biometric data stored on the smart card chip with the live biometric data captured at each transaction.

The data object (content) itself can be secured by *encryption techniques,* which enables communicating nodes to encrypt messages to prevent illegal accesses by third parties.

Authorization ensures that once a user is logged on, he/she can perform only the actions for which he/she has access rights. Under the provisions of a security policy, an authorized user is someone permitted to collect, use, disclose, or access health information. Authorized users are properly instructed on their limits and responsibilities and can be held accountable for their compliance.

It is important to note that each user performs a specific role in a given context. Indeed a user can be assigned different roles. Each role is assigned to a specific object declaring the access rights and the functions that may be triggered.

Single Sign-On

In complex systems where several components need to be accessed, it is important for the user to register only once for the entire process of interaction with the information system. Single sign-on (SSO) is the procedure that keeps track of the end-user identity when moving from one component to another.

Automatic Time-Out

Health professionals are frequently interrupted in their daily activities and may leave their workstation without proper logout. Automatic logout procedures are necessary after a predefined period of inactivity (e.g., 10 to 15 minutes) to avoid terminal use by unauthorized personnel.

Security Issues During the Communication of Health Data

Typology of Exchanges

Medical applications have become network-centric. Users have fast access to unlimited numbers of resources on local and wide area networks, as well as on the Internet. Intruders therefore have potentially unlimited access to large amounts of personal data. Three types of exchanges and accesses can be defined:

1. *Within the healthcare organization:* Information is sent across a LAN inside a single facility, or between two facilities operated by the same organization. This type of connection often is called an Intranet.
2. *From healthcare organization to healthcare organization:* Information is sent across a public network.
3. *Remote access:* A remote connection (dial-up connections and Internet access) is set up to send information to or retrieve information from an internal network or an external resource provided by an organization (e.g., a Web site).

Potential Threats and Dangers

World Wide Web (WWW) technologies hold potential dangers even if external users are deliberately not allowed to enter private networks [Halamka 1999].

Viruses

In early information systems, viruses were mainly transmitted through the distribution of infected floppy disks. Now, each time a user surfs on the Net, viruses, hostile ActiveX controls or destructive Java classes can enter the private LAN as part of a download or an attachment to an e-mail message. Most viruses are not harmful but some may cause serious damage, destroying files or performing other malicious functions. Viruses can consume disk space, memory, or CPU resources, and affect the performance of a machine. They share the common feature of acting without the user's knowledge. Types of viruses include *boot sector viruses, file infectors*, and *macro viruses* [Randall 1999]. Boot sector viruses infect the boot sector (floppy disks, hard disks), as the virus is loaded into the memory during the boot process.

The most common viruses are file infectors, also called parasitic viruses that attach themselves to executable files. They reside in memory (even when the application ends, the virus remains in memory) and when the user launches another program the virus replicates and infects that program as well.

A macro virus is found in areas where users are assisted in automating tasks through the creation of small programs called macros, as found in the Microsoft Office suite.

Other programs that fit only part of that definition are *worms, Trojan horses,* and *droppers*. A worm is a program that replicates itself without infecting other programs using the network. A Trojan horse hides in another program and is triggered when the program is launched. Droppers are programs that avoid antivirus detection by using encryption techniques and transporting viruses at the occurrence of a specific event.

Intercepting Threats

During communication on the Internet (e.g., through e-mail), messages bounce from node (server) to node on their way to the recipient, providing opportunities for interferences. During transmission, potential threats that may occur include

- *masquerade* in which a user misuses the identity of another user (message origin authentication);
- *IP spoofing* in which intruders create packets with fake IP addresses and exploit applications that use authentication based on IP;
- *missrouting;*
- *modification* of information (e.g., replacement, insertion, and deletion); and
- *packet sniffing* in which the invaders directly read confidential transmitted information including log-on information.

Message Securing

Sending a message over the Internet is like sending a postcard: anybody can read the message. Secure transactions across the Internet need specific measures based on the underlying basic principles.

Data Encryption

To avoid a third party being able to read transmitted data, the sender's original message (plain text) must be hidden by means of cryptographic algorithms known as ciphers (i.e., a mathematical formula). The process of encryption entails the transformation of data (called *plain text*) into incomprehensible data (called *ciphertext*). The transformed piece of data is called a *cryptogram*. Decryption is the reverse process. There are currently two main approaches in use: symmetric (or private key) and asymmetric (or public key) encryption (Figure 9.4).

Algorithm	Developed by	Type	Key Size	Applications
Blowfish	B. Schneier	Symmetric	32 to 448 bits	Very complex, hard-to-break algorithm. Uses large memory resources
CAST-128	C. Adams S. Tavres	Symmetric	40 to 128 bit (multiple of 8, default 128)	Used in PGP block cipher
IDEA	X. Lai J. Massey	Symmetric	128 bits	Faster and more secure than DES used in PGP. Block cipher
RC5	R. Rivest	Symmetric	0 to 65,536 (multiple of 8, default 128)	Block cipher
Diffie–Hellman	W. Diffie M. Hellman	Asymmetric	Up to 1,024 bits	Used for key exchange
DSS	NIST	Asymmetric	512 to 1,024 bits (DSA)	Digital signature-only algorithm
RSA	R. Rivest A. Shamir L. Adleman	Asymmetric	Up to 2,048 bits	Used for encryption, digital signatures, and key exchange
Triple DES	W. Diffie M. Hellman W. Tuckman	Symmetric	112 or 168 bits	DES used in PGP
DES	D. Coppersmith H. Feistel W. Tuckman	Symmetric	56 bits	Used in PGP block cipher

Figure 9.4: Overview of conventional Encryption Algorithms. IDEA—International Data Encryption Algorithm; RC—Rivest's Cipher; DES—Data Encryption Standard; DSS—Digital Signature Standard; RSA—Rivest–Shamir–Adleman

Symmetric encryption: The same key is used for both encryption and decryption. An example is the *data encryption standard* (DES) originally developed by IBM. Others are RC2, RC4, and IDEA (International Data Encryption Algorithm). The main disadvantage with this scheme is that if a third party knows the key, the security process is compromised.

Asymmetric encryption: Each user possesses a pair of keys, a private and a public key that are complementary and mathematically related. Private keys are kept secret and known only to their owners. A message encrypted with the public key of x can be decrypted only by the private key of x. Encryption and decryption keys are different. There are several popular data encryption methods in use such as the RSA (Rivest–Shamir–Adleman) and DSA (Digital Signature Algorithm). Although both private and public keys are mathematically related, the private key cannot be inferred from the public key, and the private key can decrypt messages encrypted with the corresponding public key. Asymmetric encryption has two weaknesses. First, it is necessary to find a person's public key, for example by using LDAP (Lightweight Directory Access Protocol), the Internet's directory service. Second, the approach requires high computing power and can be rather slow. Using symmetric encryption to encrypt the message content and then encrypt the key using asymmetric encryption (*digital envelope*) could solve this performance problem.

Digital Signatures

The development of electronic documents emphasizes the importance and meaning of signatures that are traditionally locked into paper-based documents [Downey 1999]. A handwritten signature expresses the writing dynamics of the author and is independent of the information content. A *digital signature* guarantees the correct authentication of the author of a message or document. It is based on asymmetric cryptography and is a function of the information content and the private key of the person signing the document (Figure 9.5).

The production of a digital signature is a two-phase process that generates an encrypted hash result. Before a message is transferred, the originator of the file compresses the file according to a special algorithm. This reduced version is a fixed-length hash result or message digest. Afterward, the message digest or hash is encrypted with the sender's private key and results in a digital signature. Together with the message, the digital signature is sent over the network. On the recipient side, the same hash function is applied to the message and compared with the decrypted hash result using the public key of the sender. Parts that match are authentic, ensuring that the message has not been tampered with during transmission.

Signing a document implies that the application enables signing capabilities. The user selects the role(s) he/she wants to include in the digital signature and verifies what needs to be signed. Verifying a document on the receiver's side implies that the application has signing capabilities, and that the key and role certificates are validated. The use of hardware tokens for system access also facilitates electronic signatures. Since possession of the token

SENDER

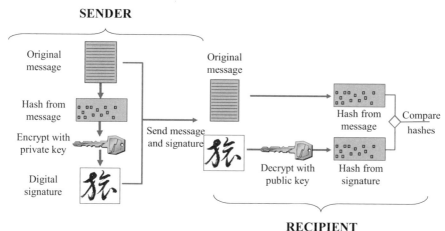

Figure 9.5: Basics of digital signatures.

authenticates the user, the token is used as the official electronic signature for signing electronic documents.

Nonrepudiation

Nonrepudiation gives a system the ability to confirm both the transmission and the reception of a message. Repudiation of submission means that at the time of submission, the senders of information are prevented from denying that they have sent a message or a document.

Nonrepudiation of receipt means that at the time of message delivery, the receiver of information is prevented from denying that he/she has received the message or document. This is an extension of a digital signature, which guarantees that a message comes from a particular person.

Public Key Repository Infrastructures

Using digital signatures and private and public keys necessitates the existence of repository infrastructures defined as *public key infrastructures* (PKIs). These infrastructure services are provided by trusted third parties (TTPs) [De Meyer 2000].

1. The *registration authority* (RA) accepts and verifies the credentials of the requester. Therefore, requesters must present themselves to the registration organization with the requested documents (e.g., ID card, passport). After approval, the request is passed on to the certification authority.
2. The *certification authority* (CA) includes the conclusion of the RA in an electronic certificate and binds attributes and/or keys to identities. It produces and revokes certificates. In practice, certification and registration functions are often done by the same organization. The certificate

is electronically signed by the CA. The signed certificate is then sent to a directory service provider.

3. *Directory services* LDAP (Lightweight Directory Access Protocol) are directories that hold publicly available certificate information and give users secure electronic keys, or certificates, to authenticate and encrypt transactions over the Internet. Certificates are needed at the time of verification of either the attribute or signature made with the private keys.

4. *Certificates* are electronic documents containing a number of statements signed by the CA. An example is the public key certificate (or attribute certificate). It is the cryptographic proof that the public key the certificate contains corresponds to the identity stamped on the same certificate according to the X.509v3 standard (a standard digital certificate format that has been a recommendation of the ITU since 1988). Another service that is normally delivered by the CA is certification management (validity period, certificate revocation, etc.).

5. *Key generation* is normally performed in a highly secured environment by the CA. The private key is normally stored in a card issued by the CA, while the public key part is bound to the ID of the key holder in a public key certificate.

6. *Card issuing and personalization* is a service often provided by the same CA authority.

Figure 9.6 summarizes the roles of the registration and certificate authorities. A subscriber, which may be an individual, a company, or any other legal entity, applies to a registration authority that checks credentials (1). The certification authority verifies the identify of the subscriber (2) and issues a digital certificate (3), signing this to certify the authenticity of the public key it contains. The certification authority publishes the certificate in a repository (4), which holds both certificates and certificate revocation lists (CRLs). When generating an electronic message, the sender signs it with a private key and sends it directly to a destination party (5). This is intended to ensure sender authenticity, message integrity, and nonrepudiation. Receiving the message, the receiver verifies it using the subscriber's public key (6), and then goes to the repository to check the validity of the sender's certificate. The repository returns the result of the status check to the receiver (7).

General Security Mechanisms

To secure existing legacy systems, multiple hardware controls can limit Internet transactions from outside the institution. Distributed (WWW) information systems can be secured at different levels. They include the protection of individual servers and applications (e.g., the restriction of connections from clients at specific IP addresses or domains, the use of names and passwords), the use of firewalls, and the securing of data channels over which sensitive data are transported.

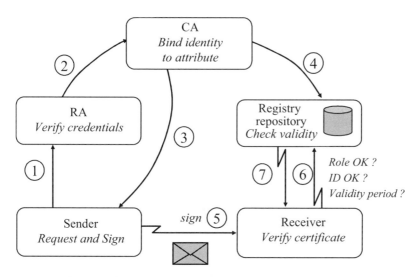

Figure 9.6: The role of registration (RA) and certificate (CA) authorities in the public key infrastructure (PKI) process.

Firewalls

A *firewall* is a security device configured by host systems (and routers), positioned between a hospital's private network and an unsecured public network. Its aim is to prevent unauthorized users from entering the internal network, to permit or prevent specified network services from operating through the firewall, to protect information from leaving the internal network, and to impose password security on authorized users. Techniques used in combination to provide firewall protection include packet filter (proxies) network address translation (NAT) and stateful inspection (a firewall technology that monitors the state of a transaction).

Secure Protocols

SSL (Secure Socket Layer) is a leading security protocol defined by Netscape. Located between the browser (or an application) and TCP/IP, it defines an interface in which a client and a server can perform data encryption via secret key encryption during the session. This assures message integrity and authentication. Upon initiation of an SSL session, the browser transmits its public key to the server so that the server can securely send a secret key to the browser. The browser and server exchange data. SSL has been merged with other protocols and authentication methods by the IETF (Internet Engineering Task Force) into a new protocol known as TLS (Transport Layer Security).

HTTP (Secure Hypertext Transport Protocol Secure) is the most important document security scheme for accessing a secure Web server. Using HTTPS in the URL instead of HTTP directs the message to a secure port number rather than the default Web port number of 80.

Virtual Private Networks (VPNs)

One of the new technology features that lets medical organizations securely extend their network services over a shared or public network is the use of VPNs (Virtual Private Networks). A VPN is a private secure connection between two machines or networks across a public network, turning the network into a simulated private WAN [Chae 1998]. A typical VPN uses the Internet as transport medium between two private networks. There are two basic VPN models: client-to-server (or client-to-site), which offers cost-efficiency, and server-to-server (or site-to-site) which, excels in security [Liebert 1999].

VPN overcomes security violations by using *tunneling*. Instead of crossing the Internet in a readable form, packets are encrypted for security and then encapsulated in IP (outer) packets by the VPN and tunneled through the Internet. On the receiver side, the operations are performed in reverse: removing IP information and decryption. Tunneling protocols are PP2P-L2TP and IPsec. IPsec is expected to become the standard for VPNs on the Internet, and unlike SSL, which provides services at layer 4 (transport protocol) of the OSI model and secures two applications, IPSec works at layer 3 (network layer) and secures everything in the network.

S/MIME Standard

To use encryption/decryption techniques, users up to now have been forced to use the same software. However, the new S/MIME (Secure/Multipurpose Internet Mail Extensions) standard for Internet e-mail provides interoperability and additional security features and makes it possible for users to use different S/MIME-compliant encryption programs.

Summary and Conclusions

The development of local and wide area networks increases the risk for computer crime or abuse. Patients are therefore more and more reluctant to see their medical and personal information accessible over the networks and the Internet. Strong security measures concerning usability, financial considerations, and the targeted level of guarantee have to be implemented. A critical element in any security policy is the identification of security threats. Threats to information systems mostly originate from insiders—86% (*Wall Street Journal* August 15, 1994). Therefore, users must accept the right of the organization to impose a policy and rules for security purposes. The organization itself is responsible for defining a corporate policy, standards and procedures that form the backbone of all information security. This corporate vulnerability assessment, covering the Intranet and Internet, is an on-going process. Actions that can be undertaken include the following:

- Physical and environmental security to safeguard against environmental hazards and access controls.
- Disaster plan and recovery: to guarantee continuous system availability.
- Personnel security since major weaknesses come from the inside.
- Training and awareness by informing users and explaining to them which precautions must be taken.

A guideline of the top ten requirements for protecting information is given in the Visa Web site. They are briefly summarized below and reflect the key security-related issues of concern:

1. Install and maintain a firewall to protect data accessible via the Internet.
2. In addition to storing encrypted surname and password information, keep security patches up to date.
3. Encrypt stored data accessible from the Internet.
4. Encrypt data sent across networks.
5. Make sure virus-checking programs are in place on all systems and are regularly updated with new releases of antivirus software.
6. Restrict access to data by "need to know."
7. Assign unique IDs to each person with computer access to data.
8. Track access to data by unique ID.
9. Don't use vendor-supplied defaults for system passwords and other security parameters.
10. Regularly test security systems and processes.

In addition, the Visa group recommends the following three best practices:

1. Screen employees with access to data.
2. Do not leave papers/diskette/computers with data unsecured.
3. Destroy data when they are no longer needed for business reasons.

References

[CEN 1999] CEN/TC 251/WG I: Health informatics - Electronic healthcare record communication - Part 3: Distribution rules. N99-042 prENV 13606-3, 1999-05-28. [http://www.centc251.org/].

[Chae 1998] Chae L. Virtual private networks. *Network Magazine.* 1998; 13(11): 21–22.

[Cohen 1997] Cohen B. *A Formal Model of Health Care Security Policy.* CENT/TC 251 WG1 N97-9. Toulouse, France; February, 1997; 20–22.

[CMA 1998] *CMA Health Information Privacy Code.* Canadian Medical Association August 15, 1998. [http://www.cma.ca/inside/policybase/1998/09-16.htm].

[De Meyer 2000] De Meyer F, De Moor GJE. Electronic signature and certification models in healthcare. In: De Moor GJE, De Clercq E, eds. *MIC–2000 proceedings*. Bruges, Belgium 2000; Kortijk, Belgium: Continuga, 2000; p. 149–159.

[DoD 1985] DoD 5200.28-STD. Department of Defense. Trusted Computer System Evaluation Criteria. December 26, 1985. [http://www.radium.ncsc.mil/tpep/library/rainbow/5200.28-STD.html].

[Downey 1999] Downey J. For whose eyes only? *PC Magazine*. 1999; 17(10): 221–222.

[Eberl 1997] Eberl U. Putting your finger on it. *Dialogue*. 1997; 8: 8–10.

[EPIC 2002] EPIC Privacy page. Threats to Medical Record Privacy. [http://www.epic.org/privacy/medical/].

[Forslund 1996] Forslund DW, Phillips RL, Kilman DG, Cook JL. Experiences with a distributed virtual patient record system. *Proc AMIA Annu Fall Symp* 1996; pp. 483–487.

[Halamka 1999] Halamka JD, Osterland C, Safran C. CareWeb, a web-based-medical record for an integrated health care delivery system. *Int J Med Inf* 1999; 54(1): 1–8.

[Iversen 1995] Iversen KR, Heimly V, Lundgren T. Implementing security in computer based patient records clinical experiences. *Medinfo*. 1995; 8 pt1: 657–660.

[King 2001] King MC, Dalton CE, Osmanoglu TE. *Security architecture: design, deployment and operations*. Berkeley, US: Osborne/McGraw-Hill, 2001.

[Liebert 1999] Liebert J. The emergence and security of virtual private networks. *Candle Comput Rep*. 1999; 21(5): 1–5.

[Randall 1999] Randall N. How viruses work. *PC Magazine*. 1999; 18(3): 211–223.

[SAIC 1998] SAIC. *Security and Risk Management for Business-to-Business Health Information Networks*. Final Report, June 1998. [A project performed for the Massachusetts Health Data Consortium and the Minnesota Health Data Institute, the Foundation for Health Care Quality. [http://www.mahealthdata.org].

[Titterington 2001] Titterington G, Bassanese P. E-business without security is not an option. *Appl Dev Trends*. 2001; 8(2): 28–33.

10

Imaging Management and Integration

With the continuous development of new invasive or non invasive imaging technologies, medical images are becoming a key component of the electronic computer-based patient record. Most recent investigation techniques produce digital images that can be printed as one would print conventional film. An inappropriate analogy of "filmless hospitals" with "paperless offices" is often made. Unlike the hardcopy of a text file, the hardcopy of a film is just one of the multiple views that can be obtained from a digital image file, and the transmission of an image file provides much more information than a still image print.

A *picture archiving and communication system* (PACS) is a subsystem of a hospital (or health) information system (HIS) whose purpose is to facilitate storing, archiving, and managing digital images and their transmission between the image producers (e.g., radiology, nuclear medicine, pathology) and requesters (i.e., the health professionals and the various medical departments).

PACSs are no longer experimental, as many vendors now offer a variety of mature usable components or even complete ready-to-install systems. The issue is not PACS or no PACS, but rather the creation of an environment where less film (instead of filmless) is used, bearing in mind that the evolution toward a complete filmless environment is a matter of years. Emerging high-bandwidth networks, high-density storage media, and intelligent broker mechanisms will foster the development of a filmless hospital and enable the seamless integration of PACSs into hospital/clinical information systems.

Medical imaging management and communication systems include the following:
- the image acquisition process,
- image storage and compression techniques,
- the image communication process,
- image visualization, and
- image manipulation and processing techniques to improve their diagnosis or prognosis functions.

These processes will briefly be explained via an analogy with biosignal processing systems. The components of an image management system that are discussed in more detail include the image filing and indexing system, the PACS/HIS interface (gateway), the workflow manager, and the communication system and viewing workstations.

Conceptual Specifications

Image Standards

The most important element of a PACS architecture is the DICOM standard (Digital Imaging and Communications in Medicine). The American College of Radiology (ACR) and the National Electrical Manufacturers Association (NEMA) compiled a standard for formatting, communicating, and storing digital images and associated HIS/RIS data (radiology information system) from the devices (such as computed tomography, magnetic resonance imaging, positron emission tomography, nuclear medicine, ultrasound, X-ray, computed radiography, digitized film, or video capture) of different suppliers. The standard refers to layers 1 to 7 of the OSI (Open System Interconnection) reference model, but is not compatible with it. The standard is both object-oriented and client-server. Clients that require services are called service class users. SCP (service class providers) refers to the server programs, while SCU (service class user) refers to the client program.

The DICOM standard has two components: image format standardization (*information object*) and image communications protocols (*service class*). Image format standards allow image data compatibility among various vendors. Image communications protocols permit the exchange of radiologic images and other medical information between computers [George 1999] and allow devices (networked printers such as laser imagers and cameras) on the network to negotiate services to be performed (e.g., store, query, retrieve, print).

Services are defined in terms of SOPs (service-object pairs). These SOPs define the service and the data on which a particular service will operate. Information objects define the core contents of medical imaging, whereas service classes define what to do with these contents. For example, the CT image information object contains items that describe the examination, calibration, patient ID, and equipment used in addition to the image pixel data.

Image Modalities

Figure 10.1 gives an overview of the evolution of diagnostic imaging techniques since 1895. At the end of the 1960s, the use of advanced computer technology gave birth to digital imaging.

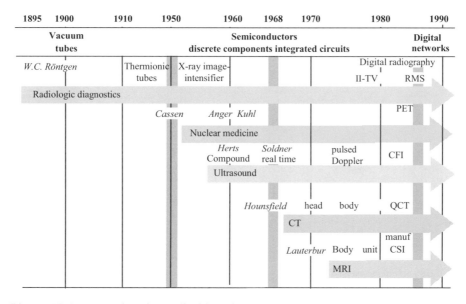

Figure 10.1: Innovations in medical imaging. Overview of the evolution since 1895. CFI—color flow imaging; CSI—chemical shift imaging; CT—computed tomography; ECT—emission computed tomography; II–TV—image intensifier–television chain; MRI—magnetic resonance imaging; PET—positron emission tomography; QCT—quantitative CT; RMS—reusable memory screen; SPECT—single photon ECT. Courtesy of E.K Brueckner, Siemens Medical Systems Erlangen.

The acquisition system is composed of sensors that convert analog signals emitted by objects into electric signals. It may be followed by a sort of analog-to-digital conversion through *analog-to-digital converters* (ADCs), transforming the analog signal into a digitized two-dimensional (2D) array of pixels (Figure 10.2). Each pixel holds a gray level, for example, in discrete values from 0 to 255.

Images can be transferred to the PACS via a DICOM standard. If no digital modality or interface is available, frame-grabbing techniques can be used. They are based on capturing the video output with a likely deterioration of the image quality. Another method exists in using high-end film digitizers. Almost every PACS needs a film digitizer to capture film or studies from other institutions. Although digitizers have the potential to deliver relatively good quality in terms of both spatial and contrast resolution, this approach seems to be less successful due to high operating costs, the time necessary to transform the digital picture, and the precautions to be taken in identifying the image.

Figure 10.3 summarizes the different methods used by digital imaging systems. Although attention has been paid to computer image generation, much of a radiology department's work load still falls into the domain of conventional images such as pulmonary x-rays or bone radiographies [Siegel 1999]. These images require a very high level of contrast and spatial resolution (see

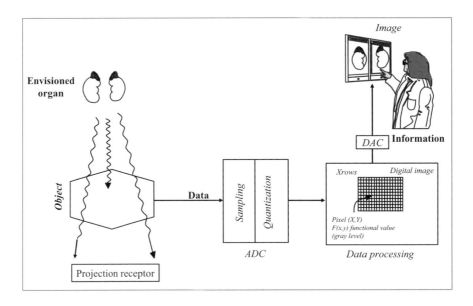

Figure 10.2: Functional diagram of a digital imaging system. In projection imaging, a 3D distribution of an object property Po (*x, y, z*) generally produces a 2D image Pp (*v, w*). Through a scanning process, this 2D distribution—after the analog output signal is converted by the ADC into a digital image signal—is sent to a computer, which stores it as a 1D set of data. The display converts the 1D set P(*t*) to a 2D image with the aid of a DAC converter.

below). Digital approaches for the acquisition of these images are computed radiography (CR), direct radiography (DR), and film digitalization.

Computed radiography (CR) is based on reusable phosphorous plates. The image on the phosphorous plate resulting from irradiation is read out as a matrix of pixels. Compared to conventional films, CR provides a high dynamic range and high contrast resolution (see above).

In the long term (5 to 10 years from now), it is expected that DR will replace CR (Figure 10.4). DR is based on the direct capture of an image using a large x-ray flat-panel detector, thus eliminating detector read out. As it is a filmless and plateless system, it has the potential—compared to CR—to increase throughput (up to 30 frames per second) and spatial resolution (at least 2000×2000).

In the development toward a digital imaging world, the expectations for mammography (spatial resolution of 4000×4000 required resulting in a 32 MB image) exceed the technologic possibilities provided by CR in terms of resolution.

Modality	Method
CT (computer tomography)	An x-ray tube spins around the patient. A series of detectors receive the x-rays as they pass through the body. The outputs of the detectors are processed by a computer, which builds up the tomographic images. Each two-dimensional image represents a cross-sectional view of the body.
MRI (magnetic resonance imaging)	A strong magnetic field around the patient causes the hydrogen atoms of the body to line up when a radiofrequency (RF) signal is transmitted. When the RF signal is off, the hydrogen atoms realign, and a small electric signal is generated. By measuring the speed and volume at which the atoms realign, the computer can display a diagnostic image. Spatial resolution is on the order of 0.5 mm or less. Contrast resolution is much greater than that of a CT scan.
US (ultrasonography)	A transducer placed in contact with the patient transmits a high-speed signal (2 to 10 MHz) through the skin. The transducer is passed over the area of interest. Scattering (based on the selective reflection of ultrasound waves from body interfaces) occurs when the pulse hits a dense object. A portion of the transmitted pulse is reflected to the surface of the skin where it is received by the transducer. The delay is measured and determines the depth of the target.
DSA (digital subtraction angiography)	Based on the principle of subtracting preinjection blood vessel images from postinjection images. Spatial resolution is low (e.g., 512×512). Contrast resolution is high.
NM (nuclear medicine)	Small quantities of a radioactive isotopes or radionuclides are administered to the patient. Measuring the distribution of radioactivity by a scintillation (gamma) camera gives an idea of the shape, dimension, and functions of the investigated organ to be obtained. Images are characterized by a low resolution (64×64 or 128×128 pixels).
CR (computed radiography)	X-rays are projected on a photostimulable phosphorus-based sensor, and the absorbed x-ray energy produces a latent image that is stored in the plate until stimulated to luminescence by laser light during the readout process. Can accommodate portable bedside examinations. Spatial resolution of CR and DR comparable but less than film, superior contrast resolution.
DR (digital radiography)	Based on direct digital acquisition of projection radiographies in which the digitalization of the x-ray signal takes place within the detector itself.

Figure 10.3: Digital modalities.

Current displays are limited to 2500×2500 pixels. Hence, to reveal all the details in a mammography, images need to be magnified or zoomed. This makes the interpretation process time consuming.

Pros	Cons
High dynamic range	Throughput (70–100 plates/hour)
Computer processing	Decreased spatial resolution (2.5 line/mm, 1/3 that of normal film)
Contrast resolution greater than with conventional film	Limited life expectancy (2 to 6000 exposures)

Figure 10.4: Pros and cons of computed radiographies.

Image Representation

Digital images are composed of a large number of pixels (or picture elements) stored in a computer memory as a matrix. Each element corresponds to one *pixel* (picture element), is labeled by its x and y coordinates, and corresponds to a numerical value (gray scale) related to the intensity of the original image at the position of the picture element. Medical images generally contain more than a million picture elements. The image processor performs manipulation and enhancement (improvement) tasks on these images. One of these tasks is windowing (contrast enhancing, gray level mapping, histogram stretching), which reassigns other gray values to certain pixels, according to a user-pre-defined map (lookup table, LUT), without affecting the original image.

The image quality is influenced by a number of variables including spatial, temporal, and contrast resolution (or dynamic range), display flicker, and postprocessing (Figure 10.5). The *spatial resolution* determines the amount of information that an image can contain. It is defined by the number of pixels per image area. It is related to the sharpness of the image and is an indication of how well two points that are close together can be distinguished.

Signal domain parameter	Biosignals	Imaging
Information unit	Sample	Pixel
Quantization	No. of bits/sample	No. of bits/pixel Contrast resolution
Sampling	No. of samples/sec. Sampling rate	No. of pixels/inch Spatial resolution

Figure 10.5: Analogy between imaging and biosignal capturing systems.

The *contrast resolution* determines the number of bits for every pixel, indicating the number of gray levels (2 to the power of the number of bits used), and provides the ability to distinguish small differences in intensity. Another often used term is *dynamic range*. With a dynamic range of 8 bits, one can determine each pixel value with an accuracy of 1 part in 256 (0.4%). With a 10-bit dynamic range, 1 part is divided in 1024 (0.1%).

The *temporal resolution* is a measure of the time necessary to create an image. If one wishes to obtain a real-time environment, a rate of 30 images per second is necessary. Some variables are related to the observer, such as environmental conditions (light), psychological factors and age.

Figure 10.6 summarizes the image characteristics for various imaging modalities of Figure 10.3.

	CT	MRI	US	NM	DSA	Digital x-ray	Film x-ray
Image matrix-size	$(256–512)^2$	256^2	$(64–128)^2$	$(64–128)^2$	512^2	1024^2	2048^2
Spatial resolution	Mod.	Low	Mod.	Low	Mod.	High	High
Contrast resolution	High	High	Low	Low	Mod.	High	Low
Radiation	Mod.	None	None	Mod.	Mod.	Low	Mod.
Cost	High	High	Mod.	Mod.	Mod.	Mod.	Low
Gray scale	12–16 bits	12–16 bits	16–32 bits	8–16 bits	8–12 bits	8–12 bits	8 bits

Figure 10.6: Image characteristics for various imaging modalities (abbreviations: same as in Figure 10.3; Mod. = Moderate). Gray-scale value for film x-ray after scanning.

In endoscopy and dermatology, conventional 24-bit true color images are used. However, the use of pseudo-color is not uncommon in medicine. Pseudo-color is also used in ultrasound to display patterns of blood flow rate and in nuclear medicine. Images of radioactive count density value are displayed using a color lookup table instead of a gray-scale table. This has the effect of increasing the dynamic range of the display. The count values are often stored with an accuracy of 12 of 16 bits, and a similar technique of windowing, as described for CT above, is used to choose the range of values to be displayed [Cen 1998].

Compression Techniques

Medical imaging entails huge quantities of data. The ever-increasing demand for more storage space and elevated transmission bandwidth enabling fast response times in a telemedicine environment continues to test the limits of disk storage and transmission bandwidth (although rapid progress in mass-storage density and network performance is being made) and exceeds at this moment the capabilities of available technologies. Therefore, compression— reducing the amount of data without losing relevant image information—is necessary to reach efficiency in data storage and communication, that is. data storage at low cost and data transmission at high speed. Data reduction is achieved by suppressing the large amount of data either by suppressing redundant data or by eliminating data outside the range of human psycho-visual perception [Karson 1995].

Data compression techniques are divided into two major groups: lossless (reversible) and lossy (irreversible) compression (Figure 10.7).

Reversible compression techniques: compression-ratio:1.5:1 to 3:1
• Decorrelation Methods
- 2D Intraframe (e.g., transform: DFT, DCT; predictive: DPCM; multiresolution)
- 2D Interframe
- 3D images
• Coding Methods
- Huffman (entropy encoding)
- Lempel–Ziv–Welch (dictionary-based)
- Arithmetic coding (entropy encoding)
- Run-length coding (RLE)
Irreversible compression techniques: compression-ratio 5:1 to 20:1
• Transform Coding:
- 2D DCT
. JPEG: based on DCT for continuous-tone still images
. CR: up to 7:1 without visible loss of relevant medical information
. MPEG: synchronization and multiplexing of video and audio
• Vector quantification
• Fractal compression
• Adaptive predictive coding schemes
• Discrete wavelet transform (DWT)

Figure 10.7: Lossless compression techniques.

Lossless compression schemes allow an exact reconstruction of the original image at the expense of a rather modest compression ratio in the range of 1.5:1 to 3:1 (Figure 10.8). In this case, the compression process can be reversed, that is, the original image can be reconstructed completely. This is called reversible or lossless compression.

Lossy compression allows gain factors between 5:1 and 20:1, but the drawback is that information is lost and that the original image cannot be reconstructed faithfully (Figure 10.9). The slowness of the (de)compression algorithms and legal issues hamper irreversible compression techniques when reducing the information content of the image. Well-known irreversible transformation methods, although computation-intensive, are the discrete cosine transform (DCT) and the fast cosine transform (FCT).

The Joint Photographic Experts Group (JPEG) of ITU (International Telecommunications Union) and ISO have defined a generally applicable compression standard and the encoding scheme for almost all continuous-tone still images. Strictly speaking, JPEG refers only to a family of compression algorithms and does not refer to a specific image file format. JPEG does not handle black-and-white (1 bit per pixel image), nor does it handle motion picture compression. The compression algorithm achieves much of its compression by exploiting the known limitations of the human eye. JPEG contains a lossless and lossy compression version. The "lossy" compression can vary the degree of losiness by adjusting compression parameters. JPEG is superior to GIF (Graphics Interchange Format) for storing full-color (full color: 24 bits/pixel – 16 million colors; 8 bits/pixel – 256 colors) or gray-scale images of realistic scenes. GIF performs significantly better on images that have only a few distinct colors, such as cartoons and line drawings.

Huffman coding	Measures the number of times each symbol in a file occurs, and uses few bits to represent the most frequently occurring symbols.
Run-length encoding (RLE)	Stores the number of strings of the same repeated symbol or pixel as one number.
Difference encoding	Instead of storing the value for one bit, the difference with respect to the value of the neighbor is stored using fewer bits. Applied in many compression algorithms.
Prediction	The value of the neighbors is used to predict the value of a pixel. What is stored is usually the difference with respect to the predicted value. Useful in lossless compression.
Filtering	Some manipulation is done with the data to allow for better compression with another technique, e.g., using difference encoding and prediction techniques.
Lempel–Ziv–Welch (LZW)	Works similarly to RLE, but uses patterns together with a lookup table instead of bytes. Works very well for text.
Entropy encoding	This is closely related to the Huffman code. The most frequently used terms of a given alphabet will be assigned the shortest codes. Arithmetic coding is an improvement of Huffman coding.
Arithmetic compression	Based on the substitution of two adjacent pixels by an average.

Figure 10.8: Lossless compression techniques.

Problems due to legal regulations have to be considered in many countries. Because of the legal and medical implications involved with compression such as possible clinical information deterioration, reversible compression is currently the accepted medical image compression technology. Many studies done in the field of medical imaging indicate that it is conceivable for medical images to be compressed to ratios of 10:1 or even higher without losing the related diagnostic quality of the images.

Particular attention must be paid to the choice of appropriate (image) compression techniques that are able to improve the efficiency of the system while maintaining relevant diagnostic information.

For primary diagnosis, only reversible techniques with no loss of resolution are suitable. For other purposes, irreversible compression techniques that do not affect the diagnostic content of the image are allowable with compression factors on the order of 5:1 to 20:1. To further improve on existing compression techniques it is necessary to

- couple image compression with knowledge-based modeling; and
- define an objective measure of image quality to be able to set a legal standard for lossy compression.

Frequency domain transforms	Fundamental component of popular lossy compression techniques. Pixel data are converted into a spatial frequency map or model. Slow changes of pixel values into one area converts these pixel data into maps of high-amplitude low frequencies, whereas very low amplitudes and high-frequency components represent sharp details.
Discrete cosine transform(ation) (DCT)	A relative of the Fourier transform and likewise gives a frequency map. This technique is lossy due to round-off errors.
Pyramids	The image (or a transformation of this image) is decomposed in a tree-like manner. Nodes will be further decomposed until they consist of a single value.
Fractal	A system of iterated functions is selected for the description of the image. Offers good compression; scaling is possible.
Discrete wavelet transform (DWT)	Uses Haar functions to code images. Is one of the most promising techniques today. Better compression ratios compared to DCT are reached because the distortions look more natural in current implementations.

Figure 10.9: Lossy compression techniques.

Image Communication System

Enterprise Networking

The importance of an adequate network and direct accessibility of images is a key issue for HIS. First, image distribution can be very demanding in terms of delivery performance for clinicians, such as in acute medical environments (ICU, emergency, etc.). Second, although most clinicians accept compressed images with reports, there will always be a number of clinicians who ask for high-quality images. So, while image production environments have a fairly constant moderate data rate where low-performance networks would be suitable, image distribution to clinicians requires high-bandwidth networks. The burst transmission of large image data sets may result in the rapid saturation and congestion of the hospital network.

Image data distribution requires high-bandwidth networks to guarantee that end-users obtain adequate response times and rapid access to distributed image archives via multimedia workstations. Networks are often multitiered and combine different bandwidths. The problems that arise when transferring studies to PACS systems is often the lack of data integration between imaging methods and clinical information from the hospital information system. Therefore, the DICOM standard (Figure10.10), has adopted the standard for basic modality work list management (MWL). The creation of an HIS-to-modality interface using a DICOM modality worklist is indeed a prerequisite to the proper synchronization of medical imaging data with other patient data.

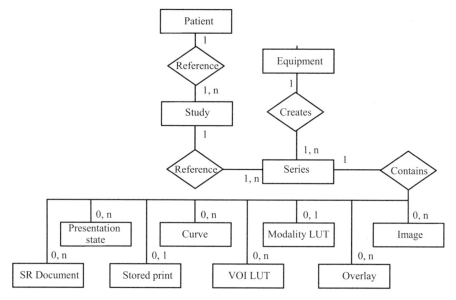

Figure 10.10: Basic DICOM information model. Rectangular boxes are entities that correspond to DICOM information object definitions (IOD), and diamond-shaped boxes are relationships. LUT—look-up table; VOI—value of interest.

To ensure that images are properly associated with the correct patient and study, the following steps must be undertaken:

- Copy patient information (ID, demographic data, etc.) and study information (accession ID, name, etc.) into the PACS.
- Enter the same data into the modality by querying the modality work list service provider. Modalities require the data before performing the study.
- Copy the same data into the image header.
- Send images to PACS using the DICOM storage service.

Intelligent PACS systems must deliver studies to the appropriate workstations (*routing*). They must file image data (*archiving*) and retrieve it in a timely fashion (*prefetching*).

HIS/PACS Interfaces

It is now clear that a PACS cannot work as a stand-alone system and that the way it is integrated into the clinical and radiologic information subsystems makes all the difference in its successful implementation. The IHE (Integrating the Healthcare Enterprise) initiative, launched in 1998 by the RSNA and HIMMS societies, tries to clarify the relationships between PACS and HIS and foster the seamless integration of multivendor systems on the top of existing standards suchs as DICOM and HL7 [Vegoda 2001, IHE 2002]. A PACS should not duplicate data already available in other systems. The clinical user needs an integrated environment: images from the PACS have to be coupled with examinations from the radiology information system (RIS), originated from the order entry domain, and accompanied by patient-demographic and medical data from the HIS (e.g., previous radiology reports, clinical diagnoses from the electronic medical record). Reentering data can cause errors and requires extra handling. Therefore, the identification of the patient with related examination data should be performed before or immediately after the acquisition of the image, on the basis of patient selection in a worklist, that is, of a name or an order number using the console belonging to the modality (specialized image station). Moreover, these data also serve as the basis of an image management strategy (i.e., the prefetching module), to be completed later on with image-related parameters such as exposure values and number of images made included in the image file.

The potential benefits of PACS reside in the ability to retrieve images based on information maintained in the HIS rather than in the PACS [Bellon 1996], and simultaneously allowing access to other data: ECG, lab results, notes, and so on. The financial justification of PACS also pushes toward the integration of a PACS within existing clinical information systems to ensure the synergy of the contributions made by both systems.

Two alternative strategies are possible here: either to develop/install both systems separately and solve the integration problem afterward, or to consider both components as parts of a global HIS. The first alternative is usually the one recommended by the manufacturer. But most PACS components are subsystems of an electronic health record system (e.g., the image and reports files). Integration involves not only requirements on the information side, with the display of images together with alphanumerical clinical patient data on a PACS workstation, but also on the function side, with the required availability in an HIS system of order entry, mailing and reporting, appointment and scheduling, and so on.

Two interfaces are involved: PACS–RIS(/HIS) and PACS–modality. The PACS–RIS(/HIS) interface (gateway) acts as an interface between the medical image management system (i.e., the PACS) and the outside world (i.e., the clinical or hospital information system – Figure 10.11). The purpose of this interface is to exchange (transform) data between dissimilar systems in real time.

The need for patient information (demographic data, order data, etc.) to flow from the HIS to PACS and for study results to move from the PACS to the HIS is an important factor [Sun 1999]. This need requires an interface to support the data mapping and translation between DICOM and a communication standard such as Health Level Seven (HL7) [HL7 2000].

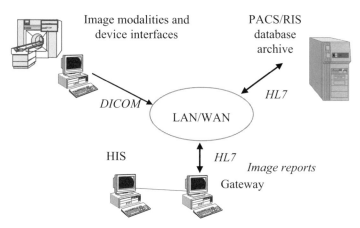

Figure 10.11: Concept of an interface engine.

Moreover, the interface has the following features:

• listens to both the HIS and PACS and responds to query/retrieve statements from the PACS;

• ensures that patient information within the PACS/RIS database(s) is correct and consistent;

• is required for making PACS workflow options function reliably;

• provides modalities with work lists;

• serves the PACS by providing (automatic) prefetching of prior exams for scheduled exams, as well as reports and clinical information for display; and

• acts as a protocol converter, talking in HL7 or a proprietary protocol within the HIS, and in DICOM with the workflow subsystem.

The modality–PACS interface should utilize the DICOM standard and must be capable of operating in both directions, transferring images from the modalities to the PACS and vice versa (Figure 10.12).

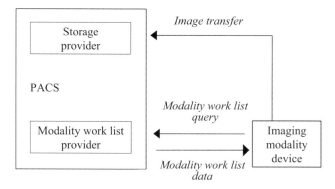

Figure 10.12: The PACS/modality interface.

Image Archive

The storage capacity needed for different image modalities is huge. Although the cost per MB constantly declines, the capabilities of today's technologies do not respond equally to the need to manage these image data in such a way that the physician can access them instantaneously. The reason is that new imaging techniques contribute to an increase in the average number of images per exam (helical scan, etc.).

The image archive is the central component of the PACS and it maintains two types of data: the image database that contains image data and the database of image characteristics (patient demographics, index data, etc.).

Image Database

The archive must comply with the DICOM standard and should accept DICOM storage (C-Store) requests as service class provider (SCP), "push" and "pull" DICOM models, direct DICOM query (C-Find) at the patient or study level, and a retrieve (C-Move or C-Get) function at the study or series level. At the physical level the archive can be centralized or distributed. Both approaches offer pros and cons in terms of scalability (ability to handle the daily storage volume), availability (recovery), and response to the expectations of different facilities. The image archive (repository system) provides tiered storage to store objects (images and all patient and demographic data) in several classes dealing with short-term, medium-term, and long-term, storage. The system manages the migration of exams between storage tiers. Most recent studies need to be accessible (nearly) instantly. Older studies are transferred to less expensive storage options (either automatically or manually). Three levels of image storage are often employed [Blume 1998]:

- RAIDs (redundant arrays of inexpensive disks) for short-term storage of active patients;
- optical juke boxes for intermediate storage; and
- DLTs (digital linear tapes) for long-term storage.

There are two types of archiving medium and long-term media: spinning media and tape media. In the first category, three options are on the market: compact disk (CD), magneto-optical disk (MOD), and digital versatile disk (DVD). CDs have limited storage capacity. MODs (up to 9.1 GB), although reliable and featuring acceptable performance levels, are expensive for long-term archival especially for large institutions. DVDs (DVD-RAM disks with 4.7GB capacity for single side disks and 9.4GB for double side disks) used within a PACS are relatively new and slow. Digital linear tape (DLT up to 100 GB) holds the most data per unit but might be prone to defects as well as drive failures.

From a cost and performance perspective, RAID ranks first, followed by MOD and DLT. In this respect, compression techniques must be considered not only as a vehicle to gain disk space but above all to shorten transfer time in domains such as teleradiology. In the future, continuous improvement of the cost/performance ratio may lead to a simplification of architectures with only two levels of archives, that is, an increased short-term capacity and a long-term but still efficient storage tier.

Servers interface all storage devices to the PACS network. Images in the (medium- and) long-term archives are not preloaded on workstations. The varying work load related to the unpredictable nature of user access to images at different times and places makes it necessary to solve the access problem by clustering:

- Modalities are defined within an architecture of clusters. Typically, image data traffic between clusters is relatively low. It is particularly through the cluster configuration that a PACS is capable of almost unlimited growth. Cluster configurations also greatly reduce the risk of the entire PACS shutting down due to a component failure.

- Images are usually archived on multiple network-based physically distributed image (DICOM) archive servers. These servers store still images as compressed files (e.g., wavelet) and digital video images as either MPEG or QuickTime and trade.

- Distribution rules (driven through in-and-out staging algorithms) may change over time. The database subsystem maps physically dispersed data to one logically centralized node.

- A browsing agent provides a common, high-level, object-oriented view of clinical events that enables the efficient retrieval of images and alphanumeric data, such as procedure reports and laboratory data.

Image Indexing Subsystem

Although the eye-catching parts of a PACS system are the archival and storage media (Figure 10.13), an important behind-the-scenes element is the indexing database that keeps track of the location and characteristics of the images. The database subsystem stores the object (image) profiles and folder structures. It collects, organizes, and manages all patient and study demographic data contained in the DICOM header files. Its function is to regard it as a system-wide table of contents/index/information server. The database system stores all study attributes (including annotation markup, window/level settings, measurements, and radiologists' comments), and keeps track of where all studies are located at all times.

Without relevant associated data, a medical image is of no value. Medical image data in the form of a multidimensional array of values can only be displayed with certain basic information about that array: number of rows and columns in each frame, number of frames, and the number representation (8-bit or 16-bit for example) for a time series of images. We can categorize associated data as follows [Cen 1998]:

- *Associated image descriptive data*: details about the real-world sample size associated with each measured value, patient orientation, and identification of the image data.

- *Associated technical data*: specify whether or not the images were derived from one or more other images. Details of other images related to this one, such as the overlay associated with this image, if present, or previously obtained results.

- *Associated clinical data*: specify the reason for which the image are required for the patient.

- *Associated medical procedure data*: focus on data dealing with the requisition (requesting physician, time, etc.) and performance of the medical imaging procedure (performing physician, films taken, etc.).

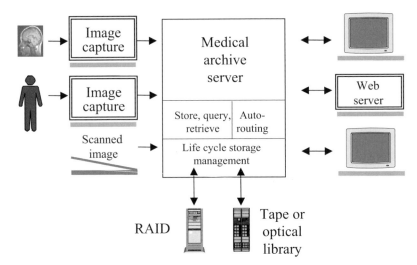

Figure 10.13: Medical archive server.

Workflow Manager

A PACS is not merely achieved by connecting a number of hardware devices. The smooth flow of images, triggered by events occurring in the HIS-RIS domain, to the location where they are needed, at the time they are needed, and displayed in the preferred manner of the clinician and/or radiologist is essential [Arenson 2000]. An important function of the PACS is therefore the workflow component that streamlines a number of processes:

- The provision of modality work lists to eliminate manual entry that is error prone, including patient demographics and contextual information such as patient location, requesting physician, related previous examinations, and access to other medical data (allergy information, medications, etc.). This is achievable only when a real-time link is available between the HIS and the PACS and the modalities giving the exam status.

- In/out staging of images between the storage tiers and the HIS based on the occurrence of certain events (admission, ambulatory contact, discharge, etc.). The aim is to proactively anticipate users' requests in order to achieve acceptable response times.
- Automatic routing of images to selected review stations. For routing, rules may be based on modality, radiology procedure, referring physician, patient location, or any combination of these. If the image is expected to be retrieved, the workflow manager evaluates the HIS data (referring medical department, previous examinations, date of the examinations, type of examinations, and admission diagnosis).
- Prefetching and routing of prior relevant exams between the image repository and review stations.

Prefetching mechanisms play a fundamental role in PACSs, offering acceptable response times by optimizing physical transport. The algorithm providing this stage-in and stage-out mechanism needs to be based on the information contained in the HIS databases (patient visits, appointments, localization, admission, specialty, etc.), and the clinical rules supplied by the hospital which define the routing needs. For images, the modality, body region and type of examination are important input parameters. Once information has been retrieved, the probability of a second retrieval within a short time is higher than before.

Digital Imaging Workstations

System Requirements

Hardware Requirements

Digital imaging workstations can be used for primary diagnosis as well as for clinical review. Studies on PACS requirements often consider that three types of imaging workstations are requested, with spatial resolutions ranging from 1000×1000 to 2000×2500 pixels and display surfaces from 17 to 21 inches:

- The *multimodality station* (specialized image station) is the interface between a dedicated acquisition unit/modality or cluster unit (CT, MRI, DSA) and the technical or medical user of this specific modality, allowing the processing of raw data and image manipulations. It must provide the functions to transmit the images to the PACS. For efficiency reasons, a two-monitor (or more) display configuration is more advisable than a single-monitor device. For CT and MRI, a two- or four-monitor configuration are recommended to hold current and previous images for comparison. Multimodality stations require a high display area (20 inches) and a high dynamic range compared to other nonmedical graphic applications. Dynamic ranges that are 10 (1024 gray levels), 12 (4096 gray levels), or 16 (65536 gray levels) bits deep are usually not supported on today's computer systems. Existing systems are commonly designed for video animation and tend to support images with a large number of colors such as 16 million colors on a 24-bit RGB (Red Green Blue) systems but only 256 gray levels.

- *High-resolution viewing stations* are designed for reviewing images as well as for the evaluation of specialized imaging modalities. Characterized with a resolution sufficient to match the diagnostic quality of conventional films, this type of workstation provides a large number of image processing and analysis tools.

- *Clinical image review stations* replace the conventional "view box" commonly used by physicians to review (remotely) film-based images. The number of interactions and manipulations required from users are usually reduced to a minimum to allow for more efficient utilization in a busy clinical environment.

User Interface Management

The user interface plays an important role in the acceptability of the PACS by increasing accessibility and convenience, leading the end-user in an evolutionary way from film-based image reading habits to digital image–based reading. The user interface serves as the integration vehicle for images and clinical data that may be located in different computer systems.

As the alternative to static user interfaces that function independently of the user and the task carried out, *adaptive user interfaces* will gain in importance. The different categories of physicians (managing radiologists, assistant radiologists, referring physicians, radiologic technicians, and physicists) have their particular needs, personal preferences, and styles that change over time.

The deployment of the Internet also provides facilities to display and manipulate medical images. By designing an appropriate tool for displaying and manipulating medical images and linking them to a browser, it is possible to use the existing Web for communicating and remotely consulting medical documents.

Although the advantage of using a Web interface resides in the common, relatively easy way that data can be presented on virtually any client computer platform, there are two considerations involved in using a Web browser. The first consideration is that the web interface is a page-based screen accessing information that is organized into pages on a server computer. Second, radiologic image viewing is a highly interactive task that puts a particular burden on the graphical user interface. With this technology, the interactivity is limited to the user indicating which page he or she wants to view, probably by activating a link in a previous page. However, this is insufficient to navigate through patient data in a multimedia clinical information system [Bellon 1997b, Verstreken 1996]. Therefore, this kind of Web interface is well suited for those applications where no extended interactivity is needed and where users primarily need to view a set of preorganized data.

The third consideration is that the images have to be converted on the fly from the DICOM format (mostly used in PACS environments) to the JPEG format for insertion in the dynamically generated HTML page. In contrast to the HTML environment, a Java viewing object (applet) can directly visualize the DICOM images of the PACS archive without prior conversion into the JPEG format.

Functional Requirements

Image Processing Facilities

There are two types of images:

- *Static image:* for conventional modalities generating large conventional x-radiographs (e.g., thorax) characterized by the huge amount of data they represent and the physical size of the image.
- *Sequences of images:* for modalities generating multiple digital images (e.g., CT, MRI, DSA) characterized by a smaller amount of data per image but the large number of image in a sequence.

Image manipulation functions	
Window width	Adjusts range of pixel bits sent to the display system
Center	Sets center of window in pixel bits
Gray scale reset	Resets window width and level settings to initially displayed values
Zoom/magnify	Maps the image into a larger area (zoom is typically by pixel replication; magnify uses pixel interpolation) Magnifies within a movable region of interest (ROI)
Gray scale invert	Reverses the pixel values in terms of gray scale
Window presets	Provides selectable presets of window width (WW) – window level (WL) combinations
Image processing	Image processing functions such as edge enhancement, histogram equalization, and application of user-defined filters could be provided through a button that brings up a menu of such functions
Undo	Function to undo the function just completed
Pixel statistics	Reports the number, mean, and standard deviation of pixels in an ROI
Measure	Provides linear, area, and angle measurements on an image
Annotate	Provides physicians with a rich way to create, view, and communicate notes on groups of images and related patient data

Figure 10.14: Display manipulation functions.

For conventional modalities, several images on light boxes are handled manually, replaced, removed, and rotated by physicians almost intuitively and with no training at all. This same functionality has to be provided by multiple workstations with a user-friendly graphical interface and fast response times (Figure 10.14).

Digital modalities generate a high number of images (slices) per study. Therefore, the user must be provided with two facilities: a "push and pull" mechanism (sequential display) to walk rapidly through the stack of images, and a panoramic overview (parallel display) of all or some slices, with the possibility of being able to select and zoom in/out on any image.

Navigational functions	
Work list	Shows a list of examinations by status (none, preliminary, reviewed, finalized or signed, referring physician reviewed)
Display folder	Shows the analog of the master jacket for each patient
Next patient (exam)	Moves to the next patient or examination on the work list
Previous patient (exam)	Moves to the prior patient or examination on the work list
Consult	Interrupts current display to display another patient
Consult remote	Displays the same study on two remote workstations and two cursors, one controlled by each workstation so that the two users may point to different areas on the image
Resume last	Returns to the previous exam interrupted by another navigation function (consult or consult remote function)
Mark as read	Changes the status of an examination as "read"
Compare	Displays for comparison and correlation purposes a prior exam of the same type
Stack view/tile view	Stack view (sequential image display in a single image frame) or tile view (images arranged in sequence but spatially separated) for cross-sectional and time-sequenced images
Cine loop view	Variable-speed display of the images to show dynamic phenomena
Rearrange/save	Functions provided to rearrange ("drag and drop") images and save the information about the rearranged images in order to display it the next time the same study is called up; it is displayed as "rearranged"

Figure 10.15: Navigational functions.

The list of functionalities offered by many vendors is constantly growing. It is precisely the responsibility of the radiologist to select what should be visualized, printed, transferred, or stored from the huge volume of digital data available and to choose the most appropriate visualization mode for the diagnosis [Hazebroucq 1997]. As it becomes increasingly common for a radiologist to produce quantitative results such as tumor volumes and delineation, it will become necessary to access different image processing services from the general reporting workstation [Bellon 1997a].

The workstations must be able to cope with images from several modalities and need to display images having different spatial and contrast resolutions depending on the modality and type of examination.

Basic display manipulation functions found on the lowest level including window/level, zoom in and zoom out (magnifying glass), invert, and rotate are necessary, but so are contrast manipulation, image improvement, quantitative measurements (length distance, area, density gray level, angular measurements), and comparisons with reference images (Figure 10.14).

Navigation functions on a higher level provide intuitive and easy to use capabilities to retrieve images from current or past radiologic studies (Figure 10.15). The location and distribution of images is derived and controlled by the HIS. Simple-image manipulation addresses the study or image as a whole (Figure 10.16).

High-level manipulation functions include tools for image segmentation, edge or contour detection, as well as multiple image measurements and transformations.

Image management functions	
Delete exam (local)	Deletes an examination from local storage
Autodelete	Automated deletion of examinations from local storage based on user-defined criteria
Mark for teaching file	Flags an examination for teaching purposes
Mark for nondeletion	Flags an examination as one not to autodelete
Redirect	Sends an examination to a particular workstation
Scrapbook	Saves selected images in a file
Print	Hardcopy printout of selected images or a whole study
Local storage statistics	Information about percentage of capacity currently used
In progress notice	Indication of progress status for time-consuming image operations (such as prefetch of an archived case)
Hanging protocol	Site- and user-customizable arrangements of images, series, etc., as defaults for initial displays
Associate report	Displays radiology report and report status

Figure 10.16: Image management functions.

Figure 10.17 gives an example of an annotated image after a segmentation process.

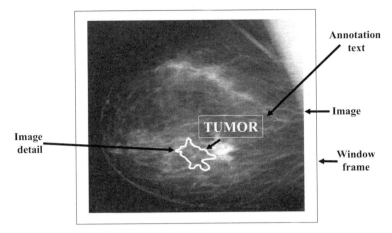

Figure 10.17: The generality of the annotation format enables rich user interaction with visual information.

3D Imaging in Clinical Use

Three-dimensional (3D) images are summations of 2D representations of a cross section of the human body, with slice thickness varying from 1 to 10 mm. The principle of 3D imaging is rather simple: images of a number of successive slices in some part of the human body are acquired digitally (through CT scan or through NMR techniques), and these images are then stacked one on top of the other. We then specify to the computer which parts from this stack have to be visible (for instance, weak tissue, skin, or bone). These data are displayed on the computer, demonstrating how the tissue would look when irradiated by a light source positioned at a certain location. A quasi-3D image is created on the screen through the effect of light and shadow. There are two approaches for visualizing medical data: volume rendering and surface rendering. Volume rendering produces 2D views by assigning color and opacity to each voxel within a volume data set. A process called casting or projection produces the views. Images can be shaded to produce a 3D impression. Surface rendering starts by identifying a region of interest by applying a segmentation algorithm. Attaching geometric primitives such as triangles or rectangles to a detected surface generates a 3D model [Adams 1998].

The image can be rotated and tilted, enabling viewing the structures from inside and outside. It is even possible to extract certain parts to study them separately or to look at the internal structure.

In the near future, the number of minimally invasive methods (endoscopy and laparoscopy) will increase as these procedures are less traumatic for patients and more economical. Up to now, 3D visualization and modeling techniques remain limited to uses for therapeutic (surgical, radiotherapy) and diagnostic (virtual endoscopy) purposes, although many benefits are offered, such as

- gain in examination time;
- more precise and improved diagnostic work based on effective visualization techniques that enhance the meaning and understanding of data by facilities offered, such as direct manipulation and rotation of the 3D object in real time;
- improved presurgical exploration and planning facilities; and
- generation of more precise computer aided design (CAD) descriptions for geometric objects.

Here are two examples of the application of 3D imaging techniques. During a stereotactic neurosurgery operation, a probe is inserted following a planned probe trajectory into an intracerebral target using a stereotactic device. Based on the registered image and atlas data, the preoperative planning phase aims to search for the optimal probe path causing minimal damage to vital organs (blood vessels or vital brain regions). Target and entry points of this planned trajectory are mapped on various images and offer facilities to inspect this trajectory under any angle.

By generating 3D models, a virtual endoscope (Figure 10.18) can be inserted through this 3D model of the area of interest and predict whether the virtual endoscope reaches the target [Eberl 1998, Kukuk 2000]. Concurrently, a small window displays a simulated image of what a real endoscope would display. A virtual endoscope could achieve the same result a real endoscope would achieve.

Summary and Conclusions

In the early implementations of PACS, the emphasis was on archiving techniques to reduce film and storage costs. Filmless hospitals are no longer of short term concern. Currently, hospitals demand better ways to manage and distribute images to provide timely care.

The focus is on maximum integration in a real-time, hospital-wide computing environment. Hence, PACS must be incorporated into clinical information systems that will drive the workflow mechanism. Moreover, the PACS system must be extendable to accommodate images from non radiologic departments such as cardiology, radiotherapy, endoscopy, dermatology, ophthalmology, and many others. In this way clinical users are offered visual integration at the level of the desktop. In fact, there is a clear move under way from a radiology PACS to enterprise-wide or community-wide image communication systems [Engelmann 2001].

By definition, archives are characterized by stability and a long life cycle, whereas PACS components tend to adopt new technologies more quickly. Enterprise-wide central digital image archives (storage area networks, network attached storage, hierarchical storage systems) offer many benefits:

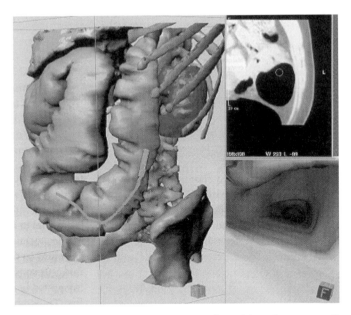

Figure 10.18: Virtual endoscopy images such as this colonoscopy (large picture) lend themselves to rapid comparison with clinical images from other modalities (upper right). Physicians can also see what the endoscope sees (lower right). Images produced at the Siemens's Corporate Research Center in Princeton, New Jersey [Eberl 1998].

they minimize the number of interfaces, reduce maintenance, and provide more efficient use. Vendors promote department-wide archives to generate new sales.

The challenge is to get current and previous medical data, including images from several experts, together at the same place, at the same time, and as quickly as possible. In the current complex patient management environment, it is not possible to read current exams without knowledge of past exams. The quality of care would surely be improved if images were where they needed to be, when they needed to be. Hence, the success of a PACS is based on two intertwined elements: workflow management (turnover time and distribution, fast and multiple access to the report along with the actual image) and integration. As for the integration of any medical environment, it becomes paramount to verify how the PACS will fit into the global organization. PACS acquisition and implementation is no longer the prerogative of just the radiology department, but by default involves the entire IS department, including the networking staff. "If the radiology department is outfitted with a prime PACS that can't interface with the radiology information system (RIS) and/or the hospital information system (HIS), you've traded a film image for an electronic one without getting much further" [Tabar 1999]. Hospital-wide image distribution cannot be seen as an afterthought.

On the technologic level, recent commercial PACS systems use a Windows desktop or a Web browser to call up images, because not every physician requires images that are a 100% faithful representation of the real object at all times. Another enabling technology that could decrease the lag time between the performance of an examination and its availability to the requesting physician—if properly used—is voice recognition for report dictation supported by a workflow mechanism.

Finally, acceptance testing must not be neglected as it is an important step in successful implementation. It includes two phases executed sequentially: technical testing and clinical testing.

References

[Arenson 2000] Arenson RL, Andriole KP, Avrin DE, Gould RG. Computers in imaging health care: now and in the future. *J Digit Imaging.* 2000; 13(4): 145–156.

[Bellon 1996] Bellon E, Feron M, Van den Bosch B, Bogaert J, Houtput, W, Verschakelen J, Lauwers P, Suetens P, Marchal G. Integrating digital ICU viewing into the global working environment. *Eur J Radiol.* 1996; 22: 221–227.

[Bellon 1997a] Bellon E, Feron M, Maes F, Van Hoe L, Delaere D, Haven F, Sunaert S, Baert AL, Marchal G, Suetens P. Evaluation of manual vs. semi-automated delineation of liver lesions on CT images. *Europ Radiol.* 1997; 7(3): 432–438.

[Bellon 1997b] Bellon E, Wauters J, Fernandez-Bayo J, Feron M, Verstreken K, Van Cleynenbreugel J, Van Den Bosch B, Desmaret M, Marchal G, Suetens P. Using WWW and JAVA for image access and interactive viewing in an integrated PACS. *Med Informatics.* 1997; 22(4): 291–300.

[Blume 1998] Blume H. The new Inturis PACS: technology, early clinical experience and work in progress. *Medicamundi (Philips).* 1998; 42(3): 29–36.

[Cen 1998] CEN/TC 251/WG IV, Brown N. *PT 4.10 Medical Multimedia and Related Interoperability Data Format. Plans - Overview rev 2.* Document N98-015 , 1998-01-16. [http://www.centc251.org/].

[Eberl 1998] Eberl U. Fantastic journey. *Research and Innovation (Siemens Technology Magazine).* 1998; 1: 26–27. [http://w4.siemens.de/FuI/en/archiv/zeitschrift/heft1_98/artikel05/].

[Engelmann 2001] Engelmann U, Schroter A, Schwab M, Meinzer HP. Reality and perspectives in teleradiology: a personal view based on personal experiences. *Int J Med Inform.* 2001; 64(2–3): 449–459.

[George 1999] George C, Sun HK, Huang D, Scalzi G. Experiences of healthcare integrated picture archiving and communications systems (PACS). *HIMSS Proc.* 1999; 2; 195–210.

[Greenes 2001] Greenes RA, Brinkley JF. Imaging systems. In: Shortliffe EH, Perreault LE, Wiederhold G, Fagan LM (eds). *Medical Informatics.* New York: Springer-Verlag, 2001; pp. 485–538.

[Hazebroucq 1997] Hazebroucq V, Bonnin A. Telemedicine in radiology. *EHTO J.* 1997; 1(5); 5–7.

[IHE 2002] HIMMS and RSNA. Integrating the Healthcare Enterprise. IHE Technical Frame Work. Revision 5.3, 3 volumes. April 1, 2002. [http://www.rsna.org/IHE/tf/ihe_tf_index.shtml].

[HL7 2000] Health Level Seven (HL7). *HL7 Version 2.4.* (Approved as an ansi standard, October 6, 2000). Ann Arbor, MI: Health Level Seven, 2000. [http://www.hl7.org/].

[Karson 1995] Karson TH, Chandra S, Morehead AJ, Stewart WJ, Nissen SE, Thomas JD. JPEG compression of digital echocardiographic images. Impact on image quality. *J Am Soc Echocardiogr.* 1995, 8: 306–308.

[Kukuk 2000] Kukuk M, Geiger B. Registration of real and virtual endoscopy - a model and image based approach. *Stud Health Technology Inform.* 2000; 70: 168–174.

[Siegel 1999] Siegel LE, Kolodner RM, eds. *Filmless Radiology.* New York: Springer-Verlag, 1999.

[Sun 1999] Sun GC, Huang HK, Scalzi G. Experiences of healthcare integrated picture archiving and communications Systems (PACS). *Proc HIMSS.* 1999; 2: 195–210.

[Tabar 1999] Tabar P. PACS: not just for radiologists. *Healthcare Informatics.* November 1999; Nov. [http://www.healthcare-informatics.com/issues/1999/11_99/nov99.htm].

[Van Cleyenbreugel 1998] Van Cleyenbreugel J, Marchal G, Suetens P. First true 3D imaging now has clinical use. *Eur Hosp Manag J.* 1998; 5(2): 42–44.

[Vegoda 2001] Vegoda P. Introducing the IHE concept. *J Healthcare Management.* 2001; 16(1): 22–24.

[Verstreken 1996] Verstreken K, Van Cleynenbreughel J, Marchal G, Naert I, Suetens P, Van Steenberghe D. Computer assisted planning of oral implant surgery: a three-dimensional approach. *Int J Oral Maxillofac Implants.* 1996; 11: 806–810.

11

AZ-VUB Clinical Information System

Rudi Van de Velde, Rony Lanssiers, Goedele Antonissen, and Vital Claeys

Department of Medical Informatics, AZ-VUB University Hospital, Brussels, Belgium

Background

AZ-VUB is the teaching hospital of the Free University of Brussels (VUB). Located on the medical campus, it opened its doors in 1977. With more than 2400 staff and over 650 beds, it is now one of the larger hospitals in Belgium. Medical activities are linked to the university education program and innovative scientific research, and as a result have created an oncology center, a center for reproductive biology, the children's hospital, and various specialized medical departments. AZ-VUB has a prominent role to play in the community. The hospital admits more than 25,000 inpatients a year, and receives over 400,000 visits in the outpatient clinic, and 40,000 in the emergency department (Figure 11.1).

Technological Environment

The goal of delivering reliable and robust software has led the institution to develop an architecture that supports the integration of components [Van de Velde 1997]. The architecture is considered an abstraction of a system's implementation. A distinction is made between three levels (conceptual, implementation, and deployment) at which component design is considered. Each level directly influences and shapes the others. At the most abstract level, the *conceptual level*, the basic shape of the solution is defined with respect to the functional (i.e., what the system must do) and nonfunctional (e.g., fault-tolerance, usability, portability, performance) requirements specified for the application domain. At the *implementation level*, the architecture defines how an object works. It specifies the structure of the data held by the object and the code needed for the operations based on a variety of technologies. Many objects may share the same implementation. An object provides a way to represent an idea, a thing, or an event. At the *deployment level*, the physical components are installed on a set of servers in a distributed architecture.

Hospital characteristics	No.
Active beds	679
Staff members	2655
Nurses	1050
Physicians	410
Number of admissions/month (mean)	2,400
One-day hospital care (% of admissions)	45%
Outpatient visits/month	37,000
Visits in the emergency department/day	150

Figure 11.1: The AZ-VUB main characteristics (estimates from second half of 2001).

The hospital's IT department was already experienced in developing complex applications. It started in the 1970s with mainframe-based applications. A two-tier client-server architecture written in C++ to run on Windows NT clients and Sun Solaris servers replaced this mainframe environment in the mid-1990s.

In 1998, a three-tier architecture replaced the original client server architectures to improve shareability and connectivity. Applications based on this multitier architecture under an in-house framework, called GENESIS, using C++ as the programming language, were developed. Client-side Java technologies based on swing classes were implemented. In 2001, the decision was made to gradually redeploy the applications under the J2EE architecture. This was based on the need for a highly scalable, extensible, and flexible infrastructure.

Business Tier

The business logic tier encapsulates the business logic of the hospital that is implemented within the information system components. The middle-tier business logic was implemented as Enterprise Java Beans (EJB) components (J2EE standard using Web logic as application server), or as CORBA objects (C++) (in the GENESIS framework) using OMG's Interface Definition Language (IDL) (Figure 11.2).

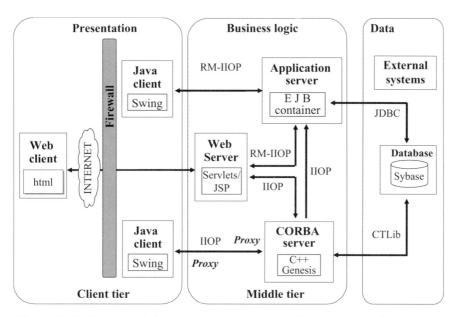

Figure 11.2: Framework for component software, or how to cut the dependencies between various components: a logical view.

GENESIS Framework

GENESIS is a homemade C++ framework addressing the business layer of a complex application software. The aim was to offer basic functionality at a very low cost. GENESIS contains a number of components, allowing a developer to implement business classes and their relationships, according to a programming model that introduces the concept of reflection in a C++ system. The framework attempts to promote good programming practices by extensively making use of the C++ standard template library and so-called design patterns, such as the observer, memento, and proxy design patterns [Gamma 1995].

A common business class ancestor with abstract relationships allows business objects to be queried for their relationships (attributes and associations) and to manipulate them in a uniform way, checking that access rights are verified, constraints evaluated, and changes propagated whenever a relationship is accessed. The actual implementation of attributes and associations resides in template code, respecting the strongly typed nature of the C++ language and promoting reuse, not only at the binary level but also at the source code level.

The GENESIS framework serves as a built-in persistence engine that allows objects to be stored not only in ordinary files but also in relational database systems. The object relational mapping process converts foreign keys into memory pointers and back, and transparently handles the mapping of associations. Ad hoc queries, expressed using classes, attributes, and association names, are translated into SQL statements containing the appropriate table and column names.

User-side, business models are accessible through a generic interface that is based on the framework's reflection mechanism and additionally supports generic method invocation. The simplicity of this interface significantly reduces the effort involved in connecting the user interface to the business model, at the expense of trading compile-time checks for run-time checks. In fact, any software system can easily integrate with a GENESIS-based system as long as the former is capable of calling ordinary C functions. CORBA based remote access classes as well as Java wrapper classes and a scripting shell are available.

J2EE Platform

The new architecture was initiated for the patient activity and resource management components using a Java 2 platform, enterprise edition (J2EE), and an application server built with the existing Sybase 12.0 database. IIOP (Internet Inter-ORB Protocol) provides interoperability between J2EE and CORBA objects implemented in C++.

The adoption of the J2EE platform was a way to continue the experience with the GENESIS project including

- a clean separation of business from presentation logic;
- standardization of the development processes; and
- creation of a services framework with generic components that could be reused in other applications.

XML is used to exchange data between various satellite feeder systems, to store data in the medical server, and to send back the appropriate information in the form of either a Java serialized object or XML documents.

Data Logic Tier

A separate layer, data access objects (DAO), is used to access the databases and other legacy systems.

Client Tier

The AZVUB system is accessible through two types of clients:

- Full-blown Java Swing clients provide high interactivity and fast user response times for heavy interactive applications. This type of client can be downloaded, installed, and updated automatically through the use of Java Web Start.
- Thin HTML clients, for GPs requiring remote (extra-firewall) access to the clinical system, provide a subset of the clinical workstation functionality through a Web browser (Web Tier).

The Web server tier is used to serve up the Web-based application and to run the Servlets/JavaServer pages (JSP) that provide dynamic interaction in the Web client. A Web browser makes a request to a Web server via HTTPs and secures all communication via SSL.

Information System Components

All applications are logically integrated around six basic common components (Figure 11.3).

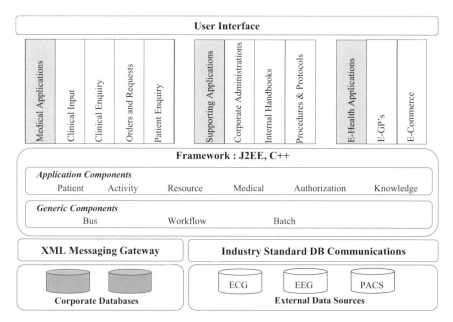

Figure 11.3: Logical view of the AZ-VUB component architecture.

Authorization Component

The interaction between a user and the clinical information system is controlled by the authorization component. This component provides a unified medium for the declaration, definition, and access rights of individual users according to legal, medical, and organizational requirements. They guarantee for each user profile:

- the security of specific data, and
- the access to a number of services requested by users based on a number of internal rules specific to the institution.

Patient Component

The patient component provides the following:

- A unified repository for storing patient identification (permanent patient identifier, temporary identifier, hospital identifier, case/contact identifier), patient demographics (e.g., insurance coverage), and patient localization.
- A number of functions for the management of such information.
- Various navigation facilities to access patient records.

Activity Component

The activity component represents the communication vehicle between the requester and the performer by managing the activities related to a patient. It includes writing patient orders electronically (medications, diagnostic procedures, etc.), scheduling and performing the activities, and finally billing them. It is linked to a clinical decision support system (as part of the knowledge component) that provides the following intelligent services:

- on the administrative level, a knowledge-based billing system;
- on the operational level, optimizing resource scheduling and managing conflicts; and
- on the medical level, real-time assistance by providing prompts and alerts based on rule-based logic.

Many approaches to writing orders are available such as fill in the blanks, templates, and complex orders. The activity component also encapsulates a unified repository of elementary and aggregated activities (e.g., protocols defined for clinical and organizational purposes), organized into taxonomies of semantic links and supporting inheritance. Consumable objects related to certain activities, or other activities triggered by the execution of certain other activities are also defined. An order is not limited to one service, but may span several clinical services or healthcare professionals.

Medical Component

Medical Records

A deletion-less central repository contains multimedia patient data covering information within the medical record. Data are also gathered from various departmental/satellite feeder systems such as ECG, EEG, and so on. As there is no physically unique electronic medical record, the medical server provides tools for clustering and presenting medical data, aggregated (grouped) in different structures according to user needs. As part of the medical server, access is also provided to bibliographic and other medical knowledge systems such as PubMed.

Medical Documents

Documents vary from highly to poorly structured [Laforest 2001]:

- *Highly structured documents* normalize every data element very precisely, giving birth to the use of form-based screens. These screens cannot be used during patient contacts as writing such documents is time consuming and a major burden for physicians, whose time is precious [Bates 1994, Shu 2001]. But they can be used in technical environments: medication prescription, lab analysis request, and so on.

- *Semistructured documents* offer more flexibility and freedom in capturing information compared to the previous type and are more suited to capturing a patient encounter. This approach is being widely adopted [Van Ginneken 1999].

- *Poorly structured documents* do not tag each information chunk, but only the paragraphs in the documents. This type of document does not allow a deep modeling of medical knowledge and does not include any conceptual representation.

The last two types of data capturing are more suited for narrative text reports. Flexibility is provided through multiple methods of data entry for users with varying experience.

At AZ-VUB, structured documents, either highly structured (questionnaires) or semistructured (paragraphs labels in a progress note or an encounter summary), are stored in a relational database in XML format. Strictly narrative reports are stored in HTML format. XML has the advantage of storing complex data in a simple structured way. Every document is composed of a number of predefined sections in a specific order. The content of some sections can be preloaded (e.g., laboratory results, radiology reports).

A combination of menu systems with tree expansions and concept-related forms on the right side of the screen are implemented. The clinical window is subdivided into two parts. The left pane represents documents in a tree structure. Each paragraph is represented as a node in the tree. At any node in the tree the content is presented in the right pane as a form. Dialogue boxes as well as free-text entries are accepted depending on the user specification.

The status of the document—draft, verified, signed, or transmitted—can be traced. When signed, a document cannot be modified further, but it can be replaced by another version.

Knowledge and Terminology Component

Depending on the domain, different knowledge bases or data bases are created: legislation and billing, organizational (i.e., activity scheduling and conflict resolution), and medical. Terminology databases, drug databases, and activity databases are also expressed as components including high level service functions.

A decision-making engine maintaining the business rules of the health-care environment is implemented and used in two distinct but interrelated areas. On the medical side, efforts have been made to use the expert system to detect adverse drug events (ADEs) and nosocomial infections in inpatients and report them in the electronic health record. The second application domain of the knowledge server relates to the billing procedure. The billing procedure is based on the Belgian social legislation system and is constantly been modified because of many legislation changes. Legislation rules are implemented and consequently trigger the appropriate billing rules, using forward and backward inference mechanisms.

To cope with the diversity of medical users, the creation and maintenance of an institution wide vocabulary to which semantic layers can be added is gradually built at an early stage of development of a component-based solution [Benesch 1997, Chute 1996]. Although we chose to use ICD-9-CM as the basis of our vocabulary server, we extended this classification to incorporate our locally preferred terminology. Specific functions were developed that assist users in introducing new medical concepts and that link them where necessary with the appropriate sections.

Resource Component

The resource component provides information to support the management activities for financial, organizational, and medical purposes. A resource is something an organization needs to obtain its objectives. A resource can be tangible or intangible. Tangible resources are medical departments, ward units, rooms, buildings, personnel, equipment, and consumables. Intangible resources are linked to the former and can be an agenda (available time slots) or the services provided.

Workflow Management

Medical care, particularly in hospitals is intrinsically a collaborative activity. Physicians do not visualize images or lab results, write orders, or do other activities in isolation. Therefore, most components described above are "workflow-enabled," integrating the system into the physicians' workflow. When an event happens, a trigger mechanism is activated notifying a person (or a group of people), for example through an automatic e-mail.

The generic workflow component delivers internal and external messages in the hospital for medical and administrative purposes (supplier orders, bills, etc.). A physician can use e-mail to send the most recent report to a consulting physician or to copy an observation and include it with a note sent to a requesting clinician. All medical documents have a status that can trigger certain events. When a document is completed, it is forwarded to the responsible physician. When signed, a document becomes final and can no longer be altered.

Deployment Architecture

The deployment architecture relies on redundant hardware (i.e., servers, diskspace, and network). Two symmetric multiprocessing computers (SMP) are configured in a high availability (HA) cluster environment. By spreading the load across multiple (2) nodes of the cluster, any properly designed application gets scalability (Figure 11.4).

Hardware	• 2 Siemens Fujitsu PrimePower 800 running under the Solaris 2.8 Operating Environment • EMC Storage Area Network (SAN)
Software	• Java 2 Platform, Enterprise Edition (J2EE) - Enterprise JavaBeans (EJBs) - Java ServerPages (JSPs); Java Servlets - Java Naming and directory Interface (JNDI) - Java Database Connectivity (JDBC) • WebLogic 7.0 • Jbuilder-Borland; GNU C++-Compiler • CORBA:ORBACUS/Orbix • RSM cluster software, Access Logic, Navisphere
Database management systems	• RDBMS: Sybase RDBMS v12.0

Figure 11.4: The AZ-VUB technology environment in 2002.

The hospital network relies on a Gigabit Ethernet. All peripherals are connected to the network via dedicated 10/100 Mbit Ethernet switches. Portable PCs are connected through IEEE803.11b wireless transmission. For high availability purposes the gigabit network is meshed with redundant links between two main (layer 3) switches. The clinical information system is connected to the university campus wide area network (VUBNET), dispersed over several geographically distant locations, which provides a gateway to the Internet.

Data may be registered or updated on the different Sybase databases as part of an on-line transaction processed through a replication server mechanism or by means of a batch-oriented staging policy [Hodge 1990]. Data staging is implemented to maintain recent data (e.g., active patients under treatment) on the short-term (ST) patient server, whereas less active data are staged out to the long-term (LT) archive server. The ST-server that contains active medical records for patients under treatment is configured in a high-availability environment, with the drawback of additional design complexity at the data level and application level.

Mobile Computing

Healthcare professionals need a tool for instant access to the patient record and to clinical reference information. There are many situations where mobility within a healthcare facility enables improved clinical care affecting patient safety. Desktop PCs in every ward unit are completed by mobile computers connected over a wireless LAN to the system for order entry purposes and access to medical data.

Nurses are equipped with personal digital assistants (PDAs) from Palm 3Com, which they use for administering medication and registering of vital signs. These data are currently communicated through a serial data communication link in an asynchronous mode. We believe that handhelds will play an important role in bringing clinicians into the e-revolution at the point of care, but they will not likely be the end of the game.

Internet Portal

An Internet portal gives referring physicians secure access to medical records through an Internet browser. This application is based on RSA token (authentication), over a HTTPS connection to provide a secured on-line access. Referring physicians have access only to validated medical data including laboratory results, radiology reports, history of patient visits, discharge letters, and so on, and reference information about their own patients.

The next step will be to make the clinical information system accept data concerning patients to provide feedback from the hospital, to request examinations, and to make appointments. Advantages for the referring physicians and GPs are that they are able to follow the course of their patients' hospitalization, and are permanently informed of their health status. In fact the referring physician becomes part of the hospital team.

Results

All inpatient and outpatient clinics use the system for near-complete coverage of reports. This includes radiology, pathology, discharge letters, surgical procedures, admission notes, and so on (Figure 11.5).

The number of medical reports (lab results, surgical procedures, admission notes, etc.) and discharge letters, monthly validated, exceeds 68,000, and the patient database captures over 3,000,000 updates a month. Most reports such as discharge letters are structured and stored in a relational database (Sybase). The results and patient discharge letters are sent on-line to referring physicians on a daily base. We generate over 130,000 orders online on a monthly base, and over 2,100 appointments are scheduled on a daily base. We count more than 2,000 active users in our hospital registered to the system in over

30 medical services. The number of concurrent users at specific moments is over 450.

HCIS use	No.
Provider order entry	
Laboratory order entries/month - Direct entry by physicians (%) - Delegate entry (%)	40,000 15% 85%
Imaging orders/month - Direct entry by physicians (%) - Delegate entry (%)	10,940 70% 30%
Drugs orders/month - Direct entry by physicians (%) - Delegate entry (%)	38,000 70% 30%
Hardware architecture	
Unix servers	6
NT servers	8
Personal computers	1400
Portable computers	75
Personal digital assistants/ward unit (= 29 beds)	40
Printers	400
Activity	
Concurrent users at 11:00 a.m.	550

Figure 11.5: AZ-VUB HCIS figures (first quarter, 2002).

Discussion and Conclusions

The availability of a full range of services and access to patient data originating from a single source—the clinical workstation (CWS) running on a variety of platforms—based on a (horizontal) component-based multitiered architecture proved to be a key factor in efficiency, scalability, usability, and user acceptance.

The component architecture, embedded in the so-called middle tier layer, enables us to implement a medical decision support system that traces drug–drug and other interactions. As the system is based on a number of common components for reusability purposes, it provides various advantages that are especially important for an academic institution: reduced training costs (less than 4 hours) and avoidance of needless integration. From the user point of view, the graphical user interface is characterized by its simplicity and uniformity. On the other hand as we aim to provide flexibility, some functions are generic and need to be adapted for each unit.

A few drawbacks have been experienced. Due to the nature of the Java programming language, the clinical workstation runs on a variety of platforms, which clearly is an advantage in a mixed hardware hospital environment but Java applications, known for their considerable demands on processing power and computer memory, require up-to-date hardware. One of the biggest challenges was to optimize the speed of the different applications in order to achieve a 1- to 2- second average response time.

When moving to a three-tier philosophy, two main difficulties stood out [Van de Velde 2000]:

- *The overall complexity*: When a problem occurs in a three- (or multi-) tier environment, the number of possible causes increases proportionately to the multiplicity of intervening pieces and connections to be checked. Learning to cope with this new complexity and to handle all these problems becomes part of the training required.

- *The lack or volatility of integration tools*: Although companies move and change, their requirements are rarely downsized, and they do not expect to lose systems management features in the process! Development and implementation projects are complicated by the lack or instability of system management tools as compared to the traditional client/server world.

As many software packages are monolithic, do not always meet the needs of organizations and are hard to integrate into existing systems, at AZ-VUB we chose to develop our own core applications. We do not suffer from "the not invented here" syndrome. If components can be affordable purchased from a vendor, if they are consistent with the architectural framework, and if they can be interfaced with the system, we do not invest in scarce programmers development time. Major vendor systems include Mitra viewer from Agfa and Coda financials.

Within a decade, the system has moved from a central system to a multitier architecture made up of semi-independent components. We adopt industry standards where they exist. We use layering to reduce complexity, and componentry to achieve scalability and flexibility. The richness of the business layer enables a smooth evolution from a data-driven to a knowledge-based organization.

Although the multitier version has been in production since September 2000, we are still refining this home-grown software. This approach demands an iterating design process in cooperation with the end-user (user-driven, user-focused design) in all phases of the project. As in many other situations, the organizational and human factors were the key issue requiring a close and constant working relationship with the user community.

Acknowledgments

Many people contributed to this ongoing project. I owe untold thanks to all the members of the Department of Medical Informatics. I also thank the hospital director, Prof. Dr. L. Tielemans. He believed in our mission, supported us all these years, and made the necessary financial resources available.

References

[Bates 1994] Bates DW, Boyle DL, Teich JM. Impact of computerized physician order entry on physician time. *Proc Annu Symp Comput Appl Med Care.* 1994; 996.

[Benesch 1997] Benesch C, Witter DM Jr, Wilder AL, Duncan PW, Samsa GP, Matchar DB. Inaccuracy of the International Classification of Diseases (ICD-9-CM) in identifying the diagnosis of ischemic cerebrovascular disease, *Neurology,* 1997; 49(3): 660–664.

[Chute 1996] Chute CG, Cohn SP, Campbell KE, Oliver DE, Campbell JR. The content coverage of clinical classifications. *JAMIA,* 1996; 3: 224–230.

[Gamma 1995] Gamma E, Helm R, Johnson R, Vlissides J. *Design Patterns, Elements of Reusable Object-Oriented Software.* Reading, Massachusetts: Addison-Wesley, 1995.

[Henry 1997] Henry SB, Morris JA, Holzemer W. Using structured text and templates to capture health status outcomes in the electronic health record. *Joint Commission J Qual Improvement.* 1997; 23(12): 667–677.

[Hodge 1990] Hodge MH. History of the TDS medical information system. In: Blum BL, Duncan K, eds. *A History of Medical Informatics.* New York: ACM Press, 1990; 328–344.

[Laforest 2001] Laforest F, Flory A. Medical record and electronic documents: a proposal. *Medinfo* 2001;10(Pt 1): 633–637.

[Lanssiers 98] Lanssiers R. *The GENESIS Project Internal Publication,* Brussels: AZ-VUB, 1998; pp. 1–22.

[Shu 2001] Shu K, Boyle D, Spurr C, Horsky J, Heiman H, O'Connor P, Lepore J, Bates DW. Comparison of time spent writing orders on paper with computerized physician order entry. *Medinfo* 2001; 10(Pt 2): 1207–1211.

[Van Ginneken 1999] Van Ginneken AM, Stam H, van Mulligen EM, de Wilde M, van Mastrigt R, van Bemmel JH. OCRCA: the versatile CPR, *Methods Inform Med.* 1999; 38(4–5): 332–338.

[Van de Velde 1997] Van de Velde R. Towards a component driven infrastructure for integrated health care systems. *Stud Health Technol Inform.* 1997; 45: 119–127.

[Van de Velde 2000] Van de Velde R. Framework for a clinical information system. *Int J Med Inform.* 2000; 57(1): 57–72.

12

HEGP Clinical Information System

Patrice Degoulet[1], Lise Marin[1], Marion Lavril[1], Christel Le Bozec[1], Elisabeth Delbecke[1], Françoise Aimé[1], Jean-Jacques Meaux[2], and Lionel Rose[3]

[1]*Medical Informatics Department, HEGP, Paris, France*
[2]*Medasys, Gif-sur-Yvette, France*
[3]*THALES Information System, Malakoff, France*

Background[1]

The Hôpital Européen Georges Pompidou (HEGP), located in southwest Paris, is one of the 39 state-owned university hospital groups of the "Assistance Publique–Hôpitaux de Paris" (AP–HP) group. HEGP officially opened in July 2000 as a replacement of three aging facilities, the Boucicaut, Broussais, and Laennec hospitals totaling 1100 beds and 4000 employees. It currently has a capacity for 825 beds, although only 725 are currently open to the public.

The hospital is organized around three major medical departments—cardiovascular, cancer, and internal medicine with an emergency center opened to a target population of 600,000 people. Some 3,100 employees including the equivalent of 1,100 registered nurses and 400 full-time equivalent physicians run the hospital.

The hospital anticipates 60,000 inpatient admissions (46,000 medical, 14,000 surgical) and 300,000 visits in the outpatient clinics annually. Observed activity in 2001, the first full year of activity, is summarized in Figure 12.1. Some 110 to 130 patients are currently examined at the emergency and trauma center per day.

When the hospital was being planned, two clear priorities emerged. The first was to develop not only the information technology (IT) infrastructure

---

[1.] Adapted from a paper presented at the IMIA WG10 meeting in Heidelberg, Germany, 2002 [Degoulet 2003]

but the entire physical aspect of the facility around the needs of patient care and to create IT solutions that would support the flow of patient care and minimize medical errors [Bates 1999, Gardner 1999]. The second priority was to provide the decision makers with medico-economic indicators to measure the efficiency of their new information and communication system.

The hospital management was faced with the challenge of building a user-friendly hospital information and communication system (HICS) giving all administrative and clinical staff access to a logically unique multimedia health record that captures each and every interaction with the institution [Dayhoff 1999, Iakovidis 1998, McDonald 1999]. Another key issue in terms of focusing on the electronic health record is the current trend for consumer empowerment, that was translated in France in a new act (March 2002) allowing patients to directly get a copy of their full medical record without going through a physician.

Main hospital characteristics	No.
Active beds	725
Nurses	1,100
Physicians (full-time equivalent)	400
Inpatient admissions/month	4,000
One-day hospital care (% of inpatient admissions)	25%
Outpatient visits/month	19,000
Visits at the emergency department/day	120

Figure 12.1: HEGP main figures (2001).

Component-Based Architecture

Component Selection Process

HEGP decided to adopt a best-of-breed approach, with focus on integration and communication between a set of predefined business components. After a phase of strategic planning in 1995 and 1996, the project was initially started in December 1996 with the publication of a European call for tenders. Nine consortia were preselected from 22 proposals and given detailed specifications (approximately 2000 pages) of the information system to be built and made available for the opening of the hospital. Preliminary extracts from the HISA model were included in the technical documentation [CEN 1997]. After a lengthy selection process (18 months) covering functional, technical, financial, and industrial criteria, a consortium driven by SYSECA, a branch of the French company Alcatel (now belonging to THALES), was selected with Hewlett Packard as the major hardware vendor and MEDASYS and PerSé Technologies as software component providers. A 5-year contract signed in April 1998 included a 24-hour-per-day 7-day-per-week guarantee on the integrated solution to be operational at the opening of the hospital.

Figure 12.2 shows the basic architecture of the target information system. The role of the prime contractor was to provide project support for the entire duration of the contract, middleware tools for the integration of the different components into a multilayered architecture, and the necessary integration and security developments.

Components were selected not only on their intrinsic capabilities and functions but also on their capacity to be integrated into the overall architecture. Basic constraints in the request for proposals were the following:

- published application program interfaces (APIs);
- external exchanges through standardized messages;
- immediate compliance, or commitment to comply, with the CCOW (Clinical Context Object Workgroup) recommendations for components involved with patient data management, currently driven by the HL7 group [HL7 2001];
- existence of import or synchronization facilities to load reference tables from a terminology/reference component;
- capacity to use an external authorization component and/or to synchronize user profile tables with an authorization component; and
- access to the detailed model of the component to allow easy access to tables through SQL queries and facilitate data integration.

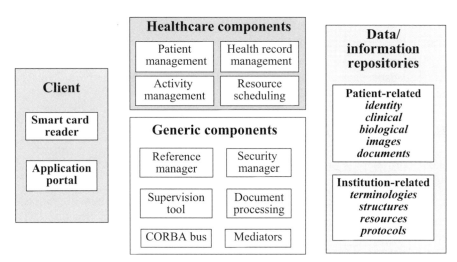

Figure 12.2: Functional architecture of the HEGP information system.

Generic Components

The THALIS-Security component (from THALES) manages the user profiles for the different health professionals entitled to access part of or the entire system's functions (see Chapter 9). Rights concern the nature of accessible functions through application components (e.g., laboratory orders, transmission reports), the geographic coverage (e.g., cardiology unit 2), and the type of data accessed (e.g., clinical notes, laboratory results). They must be individually defined but are inherited from general rights described for the different professional profiles (e.g., senior physician, registered nurse). A delegation mechanism has been developed to manage short-term use of the system (e.g., an intern on call to the emergency or intensive care unit or a physician replacement for a vacation period).

The THALIS-Reference component stores the different dictionaries of concepts and nomenclatures shared by the various components (see Chapter 7). For example, the provider order entry system shares the same dictionary of exams with the health record component, the laboratory and radiology legacy systems. The list of drugs available to the hospital is shared by the provider order entry subcomponent, the health record component, and the pharmacy legacy system.

All exchanges between components are achieved through standardized messages carried over a CORBA bus from Ionix. Exchange message syntax formats include: EDIFACT for patient transfer and laboratory orders and results, HL7 for drugs orders, and DICOM for image work lists and results.

An implementation of the CCOW/HL7 standard (see Chapter 3) allows the automatic transmission of patient context from one component to the other.

The THALIS-Supervisor is a graphical Java-based component developed to follow and optimize the transmission of messages. A persistence database of all transmitted messages facilitates the debugging of applications, the processing of rejected messages and the management of recoveries.

All workstations give access to the Microsoft Office suite and the Internet. All end-users have a personal E-mail account managed by a Microsoft Exchange server and Outlook.

Healthcare Components

Basic components provided by the main contractor or subcontractors include the following:

- MEDASYS IMS, the patient management components with functions dedicated to identification, admission, discharge, and transfer (ADT) (see Chapter 4);
- MEDASYS DxCare, which combines the functions of the activity management and health record components described in Chapter 5 and 6; and
- PerSé ONE CALL, as the resource management component with functions for appointments and scheduling (see Chapter 8).

The unique and life-long health record covers both inpatient and outpatient care. It contains administrative data, clinical data (patient history, physical exam, follow-up notes), biological results, images, nursing transmissions notes, vital signs, orders and order status, appointments and all the reports. All items of information are permanently stored (to enable change tracking) with the identification of the source of information and a time stamp. Record items cannot be deleted. Clinical information can be entered as free text, semistructured documents or standardized questionnaires. Inpatient and outpatient reports are stored as Microsoft Word documents produced by merging information extracted from the patient records, with information directly entered by the health professionals and/or dictated and transcribed by secretaries.

Activities can be prescribed as single activitiess (e.g., blood count), repeated activitiess (e.g., blood pressure control) or sets (e.g., the actions to be performed during the admission process for a coronary dilation protocol) with their time constraints. Activities and protocols are edited in the THALIS-Reference component.

Departmental Legacy Applications

Departmental applications (legacy systems) already in use in AP-HP group are maintained active in ancillary departments and integrated through message communication with the previous components. They include the following:

- MEDASYS Netlab laboratory subsystem used for biochemistry, hematology, and microbiology;
- SOPRA APIX pathology subsystem;
- SIB (Syndicat Interhospitalier de Bretagne) Phedra pharmacy subsystem;
- PHILLIPS RADOS radiology information subsystem; and
- AGFA IMPAX picture archiving and communication system (PACS) with the Web1000 image browser in the ward units.

The Information System Portal

The THALIS-Portal component from THALES is the general access interface module to the HEGP clinical information system (Figure 12.3). It displays the functions that are available to an end-user according to his/her profile. It uses a Java thin client architecture developed on top of an EJB/J2EE application server (Orbix Application Server Platform from Iona® Technology).

Access to the system is performed through a single sign-on procedure. The user identification and passwords shared by the different components are managed by the THALIS-Security component.

Several views of the same record are accessible to the health professional: by type of event (e.g., inpatient, outpatient), by department (e.g., digestive or

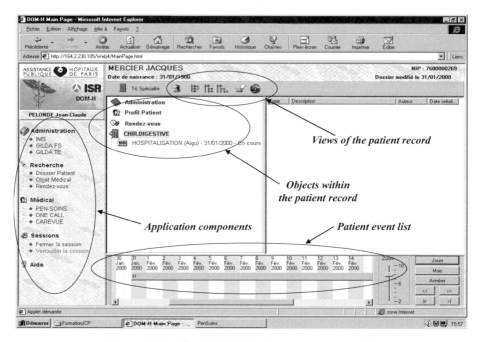

Figure 12.3: The THALES DOM-H access module.

cardiology units), or by time intervals, etc. Individual preferences follow the end-user when moving from one terminal to the user and are stored in his/her individualized profile.

Information Workflow

Figure 12.4 illustrates the workflow of information and the interaction between the various components for a complex cycle such as the imaging cycle. Imaging prescriptions are typically ordered and entered by the physicians through the DxCare provider order/entry function.

The scheduling of appointments is managed by the PerSé OneCall component. Agendas of the different providers are either open (e.g., pulmonary radiography) or closed requiring the agreement of the radiologist (e.g., MRI). They concern the different appointments at the outpatients clinics, specialist visits, and investigation planning (e.g., imaging, endoscopy, Holter). The activity component of the HISA model therefore appears as a virtual component built on top of two different vendor components, i.e. the POE component from Medasys and the OneCall resource scheduling component from PerSé. Authorization functions initially present in each application are deactivated and delegated to the THALES authorization component. The RADOS appointment module from Philips is deactivated and the corresponding functions taken in charge of by the PerSé OneCall component.

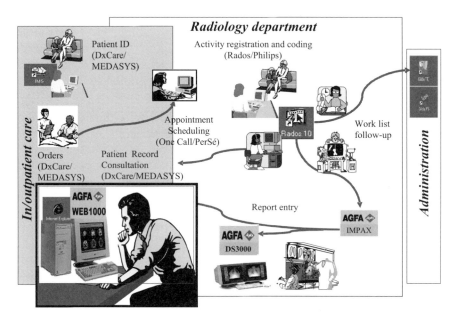

Figure 12.4: The imaging cycle.

Results

HEGP opened in July 2000 with a fleet of peripherals consisting of 1300 active fixed PCs and 350 shared printers. At the end of year 2001, there were 1500 workstations and 400 network printers installed. Over the course of 2002 a set of 200 additional PCs and 90 portable computers secured on a specially designed care cart have been deployed (Figure 12.5).

HCIS use	No.
Hardware architecture	
Unix servers	10
Windows NT servers	45
Fixed PC	1,600
Mobile PC	85
Networked printers	400
System load	
Concurrent users at 11:00 a.m.	800

Figure 12.5: HEGP HICS figures (second quarter, 2002).

The application components can be accessed from both fixed PC and wireless portable units running under the NT operating system (Figure 12.5). The application databases are managed by Hewlett Packard or SUN Unix servers, with Oracle as the main database management system. Key components rely on redundant hardware (i.e., processors, disk space, cabling, etc.). Data tables are stored on disk repositories shared by the different UNIX or NT servers (Symmetrix EMC2). Application logic is hosted by Unix or NT servers. A complete and separate environment is used for integration and test procedures.

The network relies an ATM high-speed backbone with 600 MB optic fibers connecting the servers and three distribution hubs in the hospital. Peripherals are connected through 10/100Mb Ethernet connections. Migration to Gigabit Ethernet is planned for 2002 and 2003. Laptops are connected through IEEE 803.11b wireless transmissions from Lucent Technology.

Function	No. using/No. concerned	%
Admission, Discharge, Transfer (ADT)	51/51	100%
Secretaries • In/outpatient reports	49/51	96%
Physicians • Access to laboratory data • Access to digital images (PACS) • Laboratory order entry • Radiology order entry • Routine clinical notes	51/51 51/51 48/50 48/50 7/36	100% 100% 96% 96% 19%
Nurses • Care plans • Transmissions (inpatient care) • Charts (inpatient care)	28/36 30/31 14/31	78% 97% 45%

Figure 12.6: Current use of the HIS function as a percentage of concerned healthcare units (first quarter, 2002).

The patient ADT component was operational at the opening of the hospital with 700,000 patient identifications pre-stored from the three closing hospitals. Textual reports shared in the unique common record both for inpatients and outpatients was the easiest goal to achieve with more that 90% participation of units within the first 3 months. 958 document types were registered in March 2002 in the reporting system, of which 40 are common to all the medical units. During the first half of 2002, 61,865 patient-related reports were produced and stored as permanent textual documents, including 28,142 discharge summaries for inpatient care and 27,730 letters.

Consultation by physicians of laboratory results and images was immediately available and well accepted (Figure 12.6).

At the end of the first quarter of 2002, 48 of a total of 50 concerned clinical units were using the POE functions. Direct order entry by physicians was 65% for laboratory order entry and 55% for image orders (Figure 12.7).

Deployment of wireless portable computers was considered highly effective to allow physicians to enter their orders at the bedside, consult investigation results and discuss with the patient.

HCIS use	No.
Provider order entry	
Laboratory order entries/month	50,700
- Direct entry by physicians (%)	65%
- Delegate entry (%)	35%
Imaging orders/month	10,940
- Direct entry by physicians (%)	55%
- Delegate entry (%)	45%

Figure 12.7: HEGP HICS figures (first quarter, 2002).

Discussion and Conclusions

France and many other European countries are grappling with serious problems of overcapacity at state-owned hospitals. Too many primary care hospitals and inadequate physician demography are part of the problem. The goals of building a new hospital to serve an area population of 600,000 in southwestern Paris, now the HEGP, were the following:

- reduce costs by rationalizing resources (staff, beds, infrastructure, etc.); and
- optimize the use of new technologies and effective IT implementations to deliver improved health services.

A limited budget and a tight agenda between the decision to invest on information technology and to guarantee that a relatively extensive clinical information system would be operational at the opening of the hospital made the choice of an architecture based on best-of-breed components the only achievable solution [Margulies 1990]. Despite strict criteria for selection and integration of business components, several difficulties were encountered:

- The complexity of the elaboration of the reference tables common to the different components (e.g., hospital structures, patient orders nomenclature, drug formulary) that required a strict development and testing process including
  - analysis of the needs of each concerned component;
  - use a common reference taking into account semantic mismatches;
  - development and test of the synchronization or import processes; and
  - development and test of strict updating procedures.

- The optimization of the workflow of messages between components. For example, the improvement of the output performance of a component (e.g., the production of output message from the laboratory subsystem) may generate a bottleneck on the entry of a related component (e.g., the integration of results into the patient records).
- The tuning of the entire clinical information to guarantee performance and stability.

Except for the need for extra disk capacity, the management of the persistent database of exchanged messages with the THALIS-Supervisor component was found particularly useful during all optimization and tuning phases.

Presentation heterogeneity was not found to be a limiting factor as far as the fluidity (timeliness) of transition between components from the different vendors could be achieved. This allows the temporary use of traditional interfaces giving industrial partners more flexibility in evolving towards generalized navigator-based application interfaces. Also the two necessary adaptations of the components to be compliant with the overall architecture were not difficult to achieve, i.e.,

- the deactivation of the login and authorization procedures respectively replaced by the single sign-on and the common authorization component; and
- the conformance of each component to the CCOW/HL7 standard.

HEGP opened with approximately 1000 less staff than the three closing hospitals. A very progressive hospital activity increase (through the progressive opening of health units) was the only way for professionals to appropriate new organizations and information technology. During this transition period, a high impact on computer education and staff training that started one year before the opening of the hospital was considered essential. Initial training was effected by a group of 14 trainers recruited among members of the IT department and among future end-users. A two-day training session was dispensed to every employee in the year preceding the opening of the hospital. Seven parallel sessions in classrooms spread in the three closing hospital were found necessary to deal with the heavy time schedules and constraints of health care agents. This program was completed by a four days enhanced training of 80 referent end-users for their corresponding medical units. After 24 months of activity, the induction program is now reduced to a one-day course for each nurse or secretary. A half-day presentation is now considered sufficient for new physicians such as interns or residents.

As observed elsewhere, the major challenge remains the direct use by physicians in the provider order entry (POE) system [Sittig 1994, Shu 2001, Weir 2000]. In a recent survey, Ash et al. reported that approximately one third of American hospitals used a partial or complete POE system and that only 20% of the users have a physician participation superior to 50% of the staff [Ash 2001]. A rapid increase in physician participation was observed within the first year of HEGP's operation, with a much slower increase in the following months. At the end of the fourth quarter of 2002, approximately 70% of laboratory orders and 60% of radiology orders were directly entered by physicians and a goal of 75 to 80% is targeted for 2003. The flexibility of the system to allow customizing of protocols for individual departments was considered a necessary condition for health professional participation. However, from physicians interviews, it was ascertained that further improvement is conditioned by the full deployment of portable wireless computers allowing direct entry at the bedside combined with strong incentives from the management board of the hospital.

Acknowledgments

Deployment of the Pompidou hospital information system would not have been possible without the personal involvement of the managerial board of the hospital and leading physicians. In particular, we would like to thank the hospital director, Louis Omnes, for his personal and renewed commitment.

References

[Ash 2001] Ash J, Gorman P, Lavelle M, Lyman J, Fournier L. Investigating physician order entry in the field: lessons learned in a multi-center study. *Medinfo* 2001; 10(Pt 2): 1107–1111.

[Bates 1999] Bates D, Teich J, Lee J, Seger D, Kuperman GJ, Ma'Luf N, Boyle D, Leape L. The impact of computerized order entry on medical error prevention. *JAMIA*. 1999; 6(4): 313–321.

[CEN 1997] CEN TC251. *Healthcare Information System Architecture Part 1 (HISA). Healthcare Middleware Layer.* prENV 12967-1. Brussels: CEN TC251, march 1997. [http://www.centc251.org/].

[Dayhoff 1999] Dayhoff RE, Kuzmak PM, Kirin G, Frank S. Providing a complete on-line multimedia patient record. *Proc AMIA Symp.* 1999; p. 241–245.

[Degoulet 2003] Degoulet P, Marin L, Lavril M, Le Bozec C, Delbecke E, Meaux JJ, Rose L. The HEGP component-based clinical information system. *Int J Medical Inform.* 2003; 69 (in press).

[Gadd 2000] Gadd CS, Penrod LE. Dichotomy between physicians' and patient's attitudes regarding EMR use during outpatient encounters. *Proc AMIA Symp.* 2000; 275–279.

[Gardner 1999] Gardner RM, Pryor TA, Warner HR. The HELP hospital information system: update 1998. *Int J Med Informatics.* 1999; 54: 169–182.

[HL7 2001]. *Health Level Seven Context Management Standard.* Version 1.4, May 2001 [http://www.hl7.org/special/Committees/ccow_sigvi.htm].

[Iakovidis 1998] Iakovidis I. Toward personal health record: current situation, obstacles and trends in implementation of electronic healthcare record in Europe. *Int J Medical Inform* 1998; 52: 105–115.

[Margulies 1990] Margulies D, McCallie D, Elkowitz A, Ribitzky R. An integrated hospital information system at Children's Hospital. *Proc SCAMC.* 1990; 699–703.

[McDonald 1999] McDonald C, Overhage JM, Tierney WM, et al. The Regenstrief medical record system: a quarter century experience. *Int J Med Informatics.* 1999; 54: 225–253.

[Shu 2001] Shu K, Boyle D, Spurr C, Horsky J, Heiman H, O'Connor P, Lepore J, Bates DW. Comparison of time spent writing orders on paper with computerized physician order entry. *Medinfo.* 2001; 10(Pt 2): 1207–1211.

[Sittig 1994] Sittig DF, Stead WW. Computer-based physician order entry. *JAMIA.* 1994; 1: 108–123.

[Tonnesen 1999] Tonnesen AS, LeMaistre A, Tucker D. Electronic medical record implementation barriers encountered during implementation. *Proc AMIA Symp.* 1999; 624–626.

[Weir 2000] Weir C, McCarthy C, Gohlinghorst S, Crockett R. Assessing the implementation process. *Proc AMIA Symp.* 2000; 908–912.

13

HCUG Clinical Information System

Antoine Geissbühler and Jean-Raoul Scherrer[1]

Medical Informatics Department, Geneva University Hospital, Geneva, Switzerland

Background

The Hôpital Cantonal Universitaire de Genève (HCUG) comprises a group of primary, secondary, and tertiary care facilities, employing 8000 staff members and totaling 2200 beds. There are 50,000 admissions and 450,000 outpatient visits each year (Figure 13.1). The main hospital information system in use is the Diogene system, built over a generation by the pioneering efforts of Professor Jean-Raoul Scherrer [Borst 1999, Scherrer 1997, 1998]. Developed in the 1970s in a mainframe environment, it migrated to a farm of Unix-based servers in the early 1990s. Another locally developed system, Philos, is used in smaller facilities. Since 1997, the government has funded a major effort for the integration of these hospital information systems, and for the development of an institution-wide clinical information system (CIS).

Underlying Concepts

Knowledge Management for Point-of-Care Decision Support

The main goal of the CIS is to provide information and knowledge to care providers during the care delivery process. This implies the organizational and technical instrumentation of an institution-wide knowledge management system based on the principle that the data produced by the care processes

[1] Jean-Raoul Scherrer (1932–2002) was a pioneer in the development and deployment of clinical information systems. He received in 2000 the Morris F. Collen Award of Excellence in medical informatics.

can be integrated and used to provide new knowledge, which, in turn, can influence the clinical decisions that generate actions and further data. This process is detailed in Figure 13.2.

Hospital characteristics	No.
Active beds (core hospital)	1,100
Personnel	5,500
Nurses/100 active beds	150
Physicians/100 active beds	80
Inpatient admissions/month (mean)	3,200
Outpatient visits /month	35,300
Visits at the emergency department/day	200

Figure 13.1: The HCUG main figures.

Prerequisites for this process include

- the ability of the computer-based tools to interact directly with the care providers, in order to capture the data first-hand and to maximize the impact of decision-support tools;
- institution-wide harmonization of the representation of concepts and terminologies; and

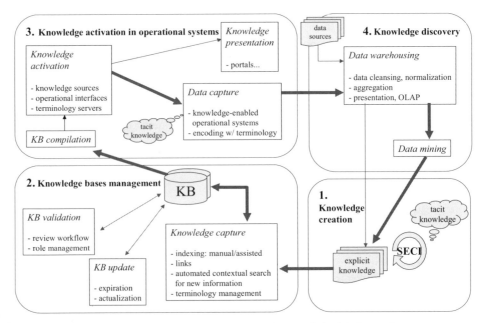

Figure 13.2: Knowledge management cycle in the clinical information system. SECI—socialization, externalization, combination, internalization (adapted from I. Nonaka [1994]).

- a strong commitment of the institution's leadership to drive and manage the organizational changes needed, as well as solid end-user buy-in.

Multiple Views of a Coherent Representation

The thousands of staff members and dozens of professions that coexist, interact, and cooperate to provide health care to patients. Each need specific views of the clinical information system, views that relate to their specific culture, workflows, and information needs.

To maximize adaptability in a rapidly evolving environment, it was decided to build these views on a common, globally coherent model, including extensive linkages between profession-specific terminologies.

Encapsulation of Legacy Systems

The usability and acceptability of the clinical information system depends on its ability to interact seamlessly with the preexisting departmental information systems. These systems evolve rapidly, often with little coordination, as they are chosen for their specific qualities, as is typical in the "best-of-breed" attitude that prevails in large academic environments.

To cope with the changing nature of the underlying informational environment, which is also aggravated by mergers and deep structural reorganizations, it is important to create a layer of interfaces that abstract the capabilities of the underlying systems and express them in a form suitable for the clinical applications.

Progressive Integration of Heterogeneous Clinical Applications

In a large hospital, there are often dozens of local, independently built clinical applications, designed for solving specific problems such as the improvement of clinical processes or clinical research. Despite their immediate advantages, these heterogeneous applications and their underlying databases present many drawbacks when considered from the institution's or the patients' perspective, as they hinder the development of hospital-wide approaches and complicate the protection of patient data.

The architecture of the clinical information system must allow for the progressive assimilation of these applications.

Distributed Expertise

Clinical and institutional expertise is the core of the clinical information system and represents its most valuable asset, which is also the most difficult to develop and maintain. The ability to share the efforts and expenses of building this expertise can be facilitated by an architecture in which each component is built and maintained separately, even by different institutions.

This model, similar to the application service provider (ASP) model, aims to distribute access to expertise rather than the expertise itself.

Architectural and Technical Choices

A component architecture is best suited for the implementation of the concepts described above, particularly in an environment where the existing industrial applications are not considered adequate in terms of openness and functioning, and where there is a long tradition of building systems, which is the case at Geneva University Hospitals [Geissbuhler 2001].

The HUG clinical information system is based on a multitier architecture (Figure 13.3). Persistence is provided by three databases: a documents database, a relational database, and an image archive (PACS).

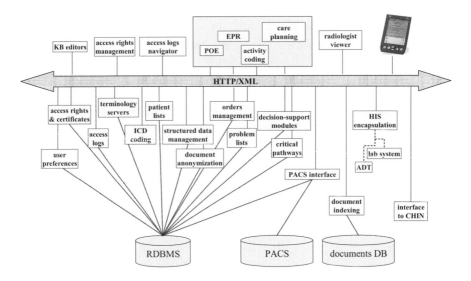

Figure 13.3: Components of the HCUG clinical information system.

There are two levels of components:

• Service components provide stateless transactions. Even though the function might be sophisticated, the whole context is passed on with the request, and no status is maintained between requests. For example, the drug information service provides drug–drug interaction checking and dose adjustment for renal functions for the medical prescription application. It also provides access to patient-level drug information for printouts generated at discharge time, and generates specific databases that can be uploaded on a personal digital assistant. The maintenance of the underlying knowledge is therefore centralized under the authority of experts (e.g., pharmacologists).

• Business logic components provide higher level functions that often imply the maintenance of session context. These components are the building blocks of the applications. For example, the logic that underlies the validation and processing of medical orders is built into a component, so that it can be used in the physician order entry application, and also in other applications such as the nurses charting system (for nurse-to-nurse or nurse-to-ancillary orders) or the outpatient documentation system (for outpatient prescription).

The functional boundaries and granularity of the components are defined on the basis of the workflow necessary for the creation and maintenance of the knowledge they encapsulate, thus facilitating the distributed management of the system's expertise.

Each component provides an XML interface and can be accessed through the HTTP transfer protocol. HTTP and XML technologies have been chosen for their easy learning curve, wide acceptance, and ability to be used over the Internet. A committee monitors the use of XML tags and enforces consistency.

On the client side, it was decided to build specific applications for each user role, instead of relying on desktop-level integration of generic client applications.

Whenever possible, applications are built in a Web application server environment (Apple's WebObjects) with the Java programming language and distributed through mainstream Web browsers. When a higher level of interactivity is needed, native applications are developed with Borland's Delphi programming language.

To facilitate the deployment of applications in a relatively heterogeneous pool of 4500 client workstations, it has been decided to limit the use of Java applets and Javascript code in the Web clients. Whenever needed, the incorporation of a Web browser inside the Delph base enables the integration of these two client-side technologies.

Main Components

Access Control Components

User authentication is based on an ID and password and is currently being supplemented by smart cards. The password-verification system is centralized in the HIS and kept in synchrony with the human resources system, so that the existence of access rights is dependent on the existence of a contract between the professional and the institution.

Access rights to the CIS are maintained outside of the specific applications and expressed with enough granularity that there is no inference necessary within the applications. Access rights are mapped to the various segments of the institution (medical services for legal responsibility, geographical care units for nursing), and their maintenance is distributed.

The identification and authorization component also generates and verifies certificates that are used for securing transactions between the components.

Access logs are centralized and normalized. All components log all requests and replies. Each log entry includes a time stamp, user ID, component ID, patient ID, error level, and specific information.

Detailed logs are used for various purposes:

- after-the-fact verification of the appropriateness of accesses: access to each document is traced, as well as modifications to the patient records;
- monitoring the behavior of users: keystroke-level logs provide insight in how the applications are used, how guidelines are followed; and
- monitoring the performance of the various components and tracing problems in an environment with multiple components and complex transactions.

Terminology and Knowledge-Based Components

Terminology services provide various kinds of access and navigation capabilities to the dictionaries used in the system. The main dictionary is a centrally maintained common list of clinical terms based on extensions of ICD-10. Other dictionaries include the International Classification of Primary Care (ICPC-2) [WONCA 1998], the Swiss drug formulary, the Anatomic Therapeutical Code (ATC) terminology, a dictionary of orderable items and order sets, as well as NANDA and other nursing care nomenclatures.

Drug databases are also expressed as components, including higher functions such as drug–drug interaction detection, and drug dosing adjustment. The aggregation of databases purchased or maintained by various experts is made transparent to higher-level components or applications.

Other components provide uniform access to user preferences, patient problem lists, and care protocols.

Document Processing Components

Natural language processing-based tools provide services for conceptual indexing, document anonymization, spell checking, and text generation from structured data. Other services include XSL-based report generation, distributed printing, and document life-cycle management.

Encapsulation of Legacy and Commercial Systems

The Picture Archiving and Communication System (PACS), which handles 10,000 new radiologic images daily, and the radiology information system

(RIS) are encapsulated and provide the services necessary for integrating radiology requests, images, and related reports in clinical applications, even though they use DICOM as the internal communication standard.

Admission discharge and transfer (ADT) functions of the two hospital information systems and master patient index functions are integrated and abstracted into a uniform interface for the clinical applications, thus shielding them from ongoing changes in the currently merging administrative systems. Results produced by the 23 laboratories of the institution are also encapsulated.

Clinical Applications

Clinical applications are built by assembling the components of the middleware layer. The flexibility of the assembly process enables the development of ergonomic, role-specific views and can be deployed on various platforms, including workstations, wireless-networked laptops, and handheld computers, while retaining the consistency of the underlying structure. Coherence in presentation and navigation is based on Web paradigms and enhanced by the use of a graphical charter developed by a professional graphic designer.

The main clinical application for physicians integrates the following capabilities: patient lists management, multiaxial navigation in the electronic patient record giving access to 2,500,000+ documents, order entry with clinical decision support, paragraph-level structured clinical notes capture, item-level structured data capture, radiologic images viewer (both JPEG and DICOM), intelligent links to MEDLINE, and other resources. This application is deployed on workstations and on wireless-networked laptop computers for use during bedside clinical rounds.

A significant effort has been put into promoting an institution-wide dictionary for clinical concepts [Breant 1999], which underlies the capture of structured information and enables its sharing and aggregation. This dictionary is centrally maintained. It is used in various applications, including questionnaires used for clinical documentation, diagnostic and procedure coding, and clinical decision-support tools.

However, not all clinical information can be structured, as this would lead to an intolerable loss of expressiveness. To structure and characterize clinical narratives, minimal levels of structure have been implemented including the typology of documents and, within each document, the structure of paragraphs [Lovis 2001]. This explicit structure of documents has several advantages. It allows the production of consolidated views of the documents for care providers, like concatenation of all history paragraphs chronologically. It is also the first step toward deeper analysis of the text, as lexical and rule-based knowledge needed to analyze various categories of medical texts can be very different. Finally, a good knowledge of document structure is of great help for automatic anonymization. Documents are stored in two formats: as sets of paragraphs linked in a relational SQL database, and as read-only viewable documents in a document management system.

The main application for nurses provides care planning and documentation capabilities based on normalized terminologies, from which the patient care work load can be derived and used for resource allocation.

More specific applications include the decentralized management of detailed access rights, diagnostic and procedure encoding by clinicians, specific views and workflows for radiologists, anesthesiologists, chemotherapy protocols prescription, chemotherapeutic agents preparation, and clinical research protocols.

The creation and maintenance of knowledge bases is a significant challenge in an institution where much of the know-how is not represented explicitly. To stimulate the various processes of knowledge management illustrated in Figure 13.2, several approaches have been used:

- The access to information present on the institution's intranet has been enhanced by role-specific search engines that can be embedded in clinical applications. The quality and accuracy of the information is verified by editorial teams, who also index the Web pages using the MeSH terminology. Information is therefore more accessible and more used, thus increasing its perceived value and adding incentives for its maintenance.

- Several hundred handheld computers [Tschopp 2001] have been distributed to staff physicians, loaded with locally built reference tools that can be updated on synchronization devices available throughout the institution. Reference tools include the Swiss drug formulary augmented with the hospital formulary, recommendations for empirical antibiotherapy based on local bacterial resistances, clinical formulas and scores, and a tool for drug dosing in renal insufficiency.

In addition, a database of local practices and recommendations can be maintained and augmented by physicians using a Web-based interface available on all clinical workstations. New information is validated on-line by designated experts, and older information is flagged for review and update. Once validated, the information is made available for synchronization on the handhelds. This application has enabled the creation of domain-specific reference tools (currently in internal medicine, pediatrics, anesthesiology, and ophthalmology), maintained mostly by interns and residents, and validated by local experts for the consistency of contents and presentation. The distribution on popular handhelds has been a major stimulus for this new type of distributed knowledge capture. The database can also be reused in other applications, for access through the intranet's search engines or within the physician order entry system.

Extension beyond the limits of the institution is still at an early stage and currently includes the exchange of patient data using a public key infrastructure (PKI) based secure e-mail as well as teleradiology services and neurosurgical advice to neighboring hospitals. Remote access to components of the clinical information system over the Internet is currently being experimented by another Swiss university hospital and with Geneva community physicians.

Results

Figure 13.4 summarizes the mains characteristics and use figures for the clinical information system. More than 700 users in 40 medical services use the documentation system at HCUG, mostly for the transcription of dictated reports. All inpatient clinics are using the system for a coverage exceeding 80% of official reports. This includes radiology reports, pathology reports, surgical procedures, and discharge letters among others, but not progress notes, which can be captured directly by clinicians in the electronic patient record. Most medical outpatient clinics are in the process of using the system for patient summaries and discharge reports.

	No.
Patient order entry	
Laboratory order entries/month - Direct entry by physicians (%) - Delegate entry (nurses, clerks) (%)	80,000 30% 70%
Image orders /month - Direct entry by physicians (%) - Delegate entry (nurses, clerks) (%)	9,000 0% 100%
Drug orders/month - Direct entry by physicians (%) - Delegate entry (nurses, clerks) (%)	2 pilot units only 100% 0%
Hardware architecture	
Unix servers	70
Window servers	20
PC, portable computers	4,500
Personal digital assistants/100 active beds	500
Printers	800

Figure 13.4: HCUG figures (second semester, 2001).

Discussion and Conclusions

As the various applications are being deployed and appropriated by the users, there is a need for the development of additional views and the implementation of more complex collaborative workflows. The boundaries between clinical and administrative applications tend to become blurred, thus mandating transversal, institution-wide approaches for the implementation of resource scheduling, and messaging functions.

Modeling of multidisciplinary guidelines and care pathways, and their implementation into the order entry, resource scheduling, event handling, and notification components is a key area of development as the potential use of these systems for the improvement of the quality and efficacy of care processes becomes clear.

References

[Breant 1999] Breant C, Borst F, Campi D, Griesser V, Momjian S. A hospital-wide clinical findings dictionary based on an extension of the International Classification of Diseases (ICD). *Proc AMIA Symp.* 1999; 706–710.

[Borst 1999] Borst F, Appel R, Baud R, Ligier Y, Scherrer JR. Happy birthday DIOGENE: a hospital information system born 20 years ago. *Int J Med Inform.* 1999; 54(3): 157–167.

[Geissbuhler 2001] Geissbuhler A, Lovis C, Lamb A, Spahni S. Experience with an XML/HTTP-based federative approach to develop a hospital-wide clinical information system. *Medinfo.* 2001;10(Pt 1): 735–739.

[Lovis 2001] Lovis C, Baud R, Revillard C, Pult L, Borst F, Geissbuhler A. Paragraph-oriented structure for narratives in medical documentation. *Medinfo.* 2001; 638–642.

[Nonaka 1994) Nonaka I. A Dynamic Theory of Organizational Knowledge Creation, *Organization Science 1994;* 5: 14–37.

[Scherrer 1997] Scherrer JR, Lovis C, Baud R, Borst F. Integrated computerized patient records: the Diogene 2 distributed architecture paradigm with special emphasis on its middleware design. In: Iakovidis I, Maglavera S, Trakatellis A, eds. *User Acceptance of Health Telematics Applications, Looking for Convincing Cases.* Amsterdam: IOS Press, 1998; 15–31.

[Scherrer 1998] Scherrer JR, Lovis C, Baud R, Borst F, Spahni S. Integrated computerized patient records: the DIOGENE 2 distributed architecture paradigm with special emphasis on its middleware design. *Stud Health Technol Inform* 1998; 56: 15–31.

[Tschopp 2001] Tschopp M, Geissbuhler A. Use of handheld computers as bedside information providers. *Medinfo 2001*; 764–767.

[WONCA 1998] World Organization of Family Doctors, WONCA. *ICPC-2 – International Classification of Primary Care , 2nd edition.* Oxford Medical Publications, 1998.

14

VUMC Clinical Information System

William W. Stead, Randall A. Bates, Jeff Byrd, Dario Giuse, Randolph A. Miller, and Edward K. Shultz

Informatics Center, Vanderbilt University Medical Center, Nashville, Tennessee, USA

Background

Vanderbilt University Medical Center (VUMC) began to create an integrated advanced information management system (IAIMS) in 1991, when Dr. William Stead arrived to become the associate vice chancellor and director of the new Informatics Center at Vanderbilt, and brought with him more than a decade of relevant informatics and IAIMS experiences [Stead 1991a,b]. Prior to 1991, Vanderbilt's strategy had been to select and deploy individual "best of class" information systems for admission/discharge/transfer and billing, dietary, materials management, pharmacy, laboratory, and radiology. These systems were used primarily to automate tasks. Admitting and discharge data were exchanged through an interface engine to minimize redundant data entry. A limited database of billing data supported management decisions.

The VUMC IAIMS vision was to bring together people, data, knowledge, and tools at the place and time decisions were to be made. The goal of using tools to leverage data and knowledge for decision support represented a major shift from the prior focus on automation of tasks. The shift led to three critical early decisions [Stead 1996]. The first was to invest in faculty in biomedical informatics, as a new primary academic discipline to conduct research and develop manpower, and to translate the IAIMS vision into practice. The second decision was to create a novel organizational structure, the Informatics Center, to manage information as a shared resource, and to use VUMC's operational infrastructure as a laboratory to discover optimal interactions of people, process, and technology. The third decision was to design an information architecture to manage information resources as enterprise assets separate from the applications that automate processes.

VUMC is an integral part of Vanderbilt University, which is composed of ten schools (the College of Arts and Science, Graduate School, Blair School of Music, Divinity School, School of Engineering, School of Law, School of Medicine, School of Nursing, Owen Graduate School of Management, and Peabody College, Vanderbilt's School of Education), a public policy institute, the medical center's clinical facilities, and the Freedom Forum First Amendment Center. The university in 2001–2002 has a faculty of more than 1900 full-time faculty members; a part-time and clinical faculty of approximately 1500; and a staff of almost 12,600. Undergraduate students number 6037 and there are 4157 graduate and professional students.

VUMC's clinical facilities include the 678-bed Vanderbilt University Hospital (VUH), an 88-bed Psychiatric Hospital, the 75-bed Vanderbilt Stallworth Rehabilitation Hospital, and outpatient facilities in the Vanderbilt Clinic (TVC). Operating statistics for VUH and TVC for Fiscal Year 2001 are listed in Figure 14.1.

Main hospital characteristics	No.
Staffed beds	678
VUH FTE/adjusted occupied beds	5.6
TVC FTE/400 visits	4.3
Inpatient discharges/month (mean)	2,657
Case mix index	1.75
Mean length of stay (days)	5.3
Outpatient surgeries/month	1,098
Outpatient visits/month	53,482
Visits to emergency department/day	175

Figure 14.1: VUH and TVC operating statistics (2001).

This case report describes the state of information management and utilization at VUMC a decade after these beginnings. It presents the architecture that has evolved and summarizes the functionality that has been developed, together with the impact of both upon the enterprise.

VUMC Information Management Architecture

An information technology architecture defines the philosophy underlying system development and maintenance, the components of a system, the boundaries of the components, and the communication among them. An architecture uses layering to reduce complexity, and modularity to increase flexibility while localizing change. Client-server configurations, mechanisms for mediation among clients and servers, and object-oriented programming are examples of architectural strategies that increase interoperability and reuse; they are tools, not architectures per se. Such tools meet their objectives as long as all software is developed consistently with the overall architectural approach. However, to date, no single approach to developing applications has been adequate to support all of the information handling needs of a complex enterprise. Even if one could accomplish this, the success would be short lived as inevitable computer science advances produce better approaches that are incompatible with past implementations. Accordingly, such strategies are best categorized as *application component architectures* to denote their limited scope.

Each application, or suite of applications developed for a common application component architecture, is a discrete unit. It can have its own data model, business rules, and database. When more than one application component architecture is required by an enterprise, the increase in functionality comes at the price of potentially redundant implementation and maintenance burdens, potentially inconsistent definitions of content across applications or application suites, and the inability to resolve such discrepancies. Interface standards can reduce the problem but cannot solve it unless the meaning of messages exchanged is explicit and independent of the sending and receiving systems. At the existing state of the art, an interface is merely a path between systems. Each receiving system must be programmed individually to be able to appropriately interpret data elements from each sending system and to integrate and utilize the external information in the context of its internal environment. When each participating system manages its database independently, there is no way to ensure they are synchronized. In other words, a collection of databases underpinning interfaced applications does not equal, and can never exceed, the sum of the parts.

Enterprise Information Architecture

Architecture Principles

VUMC specified an enterprise information architecture to separate the management of corporate information assets, such as data definitions, business rules, and patient data, from the transaction processing systems that support operations. The enterprise architecture also encompasses important philosophical principles, such as the following:

1. Do not develop components that are not consistent with the ideal architectural configuration unless there is a viable known path that will go from the developed state to the ideal state in a reasonable amount of time.
2. Do not devote scarce developmental resources to build an information resource or a software program that could be affordably purchased in the commercial marketplace.
3. All electronic clinical information exchange at VUMC will be routed

through the generic interface engine (GIE). Data transfer among applications is managed proactively at the enterprise level (via the GIE), ensuring the degree of synchronization appropriate to the logical unit of work.

From the beginning, it has not been practical to stop and rebuild the VUMC applications and infrastructure to match the idealized information architecture. As noted above, the information architecture specification serves as a planning tool, guiding each successive implementation to approximate its principles to the degree possible.

Figure 14.2 is a logical view of the VUMC information architecture. It permits vendor applications and locally developed informatics tools to operate as components supported by a shared set of information resources and repositories.

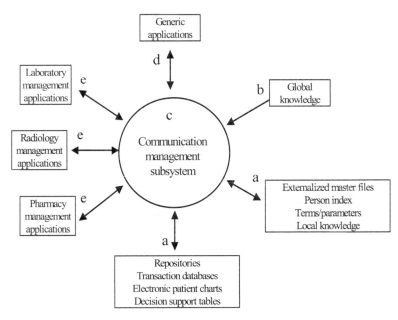

Figure 14.2: Logical view of VUMC information architecture.
(a) Enterprise information assets are maintained in externalized master files and repositories. (b) Global knowledge resources are linked in via the Internet. (c) Access to and update of repositories and logical unit of work are managed via a communication subsystem. (d) Generic applications support functions such as patient look-up, ordering, reporting, and escalation across the enterprise. (e) Niche applications are prealigned and reduced to components to support departmental workflow.

The purpose of the VUMC *enterprise information architecture* is to separate the management of content from the applications or tools that provide functionality for users. A key tenet of the architecture is to represent meaningful VUMC content outside of the various application systems, and to align the applications by importing and using this externally defined content in a standard manner throughout. Information, such as metadata and organizational knowledge that might otherwise be entered into application-specific master files, is externalized in generalized tables. This information is structured to make its meaning explicit and accessible; for example, external tables store the identity of medical center personnel with mapping to their roles; clinically meaningful orderables are stored externally, with mapping to the administrative equivalents in individual ancillary systems; and the set of clinical concepts that can be measured in the laboratory is stored externally, with mapping to the various billing codes associated with each concept in ancillary systems.

Certain applications can use these externalized tables directly. It is often necessary to manually copy the information into the profiles of legacy systems. In either case, each new application reuses prior definitional work. Only newly required information needs to be added to the generalized tables, and the relation of such new information to existing information can be made explicit as it is added. This approach saves implementation time while pre-aligning meaning across otherwise disparate applications.

Generalized Repositories

Similarly, data that are captured or managed by an application, but that are used by more than one application, are externalized into generalized repositories. A set of disparate repositories exploit the strengths of their respective technologies. For example, highly structured, coded clinical data are represented in relational tables, and in contrast, an indexed text repository, organized according to a document paradigm, provides a single logical source for all clinical reports about a patient, be they binary data, images, or text. Some reports are stored in this repository as symbolic links (e.g., links from textual radiology reports to their corresponding images in the picture archiving and communication systems), whereas others are copied directly from primary sources and stored directly in the repository, as in the case of ECGs.

The indexed text repository is a nonrelational, hyper-indexed database implemented in Perl on a distributed processing system. The lowest tier, known as the Star layer, implements distributed processing, queue-based transaction processing, process control and monitoring, and interprocess communication. The database layer, known as StarChart, implements permanent data storage, automatic replication across servers in different geographic locations, and conversion of clinical data from all sources into a common internal representation. Common views such as the assembly of documents and data related to a patient into a browsable electronic chart are cached to reduce search demands. The application layer implements transaction and business logic, such as the handling of corrections and updates in stored documents, and the handling of different evolving stages of individual data items (from pending to preliminary to final to corrected report, for example). This layer is shared by all applications that use the repository, and hence provides the single place where transaction and business logic is maintained and applied. It provides request broker functionality to support application interface services, report distribution services, and a number of Web-based interfaces.

The externalized repositories leverage database techniques to solve a class of problems that are difficult to handle through data processing strategies characteristic of transaction processing systems. For example, a common approach to an enterprise master patient index involves recording each facility caring for a patient, and, for each facility, the patient's medical record number. When a facility issues a duplicate number in error, a complicated process is used to reconcile and merge the records. One of the VUMC repositories is the enterprise patient index, a table of identifying numbers, a table of names, and linkages of those numbers and names. As mistakes are made and corrected, linkages are updated. An SQL query is all that is needed to assemble all record fragments for a patient.

In addition, the externalized application-independent repositories serve two types of middleware function. First, when an application combines two concepts into one variable, the meaning can be decomposed into a set of granular data on the way into the repository, or assembled from multiple data on the way back into the application. In this fashion, required translation is limited to a "plug-in" between the application and the repository without burdening other applications. As applications converge around common metadata, the plug-ins are removed. Difference in the use of the concept of case, encounter, and visit among applications is a simple example of how it is helpful to clear up any ambiguities in the repository. Second, when two different processes provide different views of a related datum, those views can be represented side by side instead of selecting one or the other. For example, the admitting office may be responsible for updating the attending physician field that is used for billing purposes, whereas the clinical care team on the patient's ward may represent the most reliable source of this information. However, the ward team does not have the admitting office's understanding of the correct timing of recording changes to comply with billing requirements. The solution is to record both views of the data (administrative and clinical versions of attending physician, and to have a process for reconciling differences just before midnight, the deadline for billing corrections).

The Generic Interface Engine

Application components connect to the collective externalized tables and repositories through a single logical point, serviced by communication management engines. The GIE utilizes IBM's CICS as a transaction-processing environment. The GIE provides transaction logging, protocol conversion, one to many routing, and request broker functionality. It uses queuing mechanisms to loosely couple interapplication communication. At the same time, it manages acknowledgments so as to ensure serialization and a logical unit of work across components. Since the proactive end-to-end management of interface transactions provided by the GIE requires application-specific development, a commercial interface engine provides an alternative path for less demanding situations. In addition, efficient query services provide applications with access to some commonly used repositories for transactions that do not result in updates.

Components of the Clinical Information System

Whenever possible, common tools provide generic functionality across the enterprise. A clinical workstation (CWS) desktop is used for shared devices in high-volume clinical areas. The CWS is "locked down" to minimize support problems and enables use of tools such as ZenWorks to distribute updates from a central management point. It includes an authentication service that enables users to sign on once to the CWS, which in turn signs them into the applications they select, avoiding the time required to sign on to multiple independent applications.

WizOrder (developed at VUMC [Geissbuhler 1996] and marketed by McKesson as Horizon Expert Orders) is the clinical decision support and order capture interface for the inpatient services. Through order sets, protocols, and guidelines developed and maintained by local clinical experts (who utilize the literature and national guidelines), WizOrder brings together information about the patient with information about best practices appropriate to the clinical context. As the provider makes decisions in this supportive environment, WizOrder translates them into actionable orders, which are in turn distributed as appropriate by the GIE.

PathworX is another tool linking pathway management, standardized nursing documentation, and variance tracking [Ozbolt 1996]. PathworX enables customized implementation of best-practice care protocols, cuing caregivers to perform and document needed services. By tracking variances in achievement of therapeutic goals, PathworX identifies the services at particular phases of particular pathways that were less effective than anticipated. Goal variance data support the generation and testing of hypotheses for continual quality improvement.

Web-based interfaces to StarChart [Giuse 1996] provide access to the electronic patient chart and support for related workflow. A one-patient-at-a-time interface provides access to the integrated clinical picture for one patient. A panel management or practice-oriented interface allows entire sets of patients to be accessed and reviewed in a single logical operation, and includes a result notification component. A number of additional interfaces are used for data entry, validation, document submission, document signature, report generation, and ad hoc querying.

To facilitate rapid development, a general set of services is made available. Due to different client needs, sometimes multiple methods are available to access the same service (e.g., Java RMI, HTTP, CORBA). All these access methods call the same code, however. Representative services include the following:

- *Enterprise Patient Identifier Service*: Data include additional fields such as Social Security number, date of birth, and address information. Increase query functionality by supporting queries with multiple partial fields (e.g., partial name and medical record number).

- *Census Service*:

    - Inpatient—Service to query inpatient census information by location.

    - Outpatient—Service to query outpatient census information by location, attending, medical record number, and patient name.

- *DocInfo, Enterprise Java Beans (EJB)*: Service to allow clients to query physician information using a variety of parameters (name, sign on, resource ID).

- *Orderable Finder*: Service providing a route to identify what clinical items/functions can be ordered.

- *ICD Finder*: Searches ICD-9 code for a diagnosis.

- *Compliance Information Service*: Matches CPT (Current Procedure Terminology) to Medicare compliant ICD.

- *Medication Look-up*: Service to allow look-up of a medication, potential doses, routes, and frequencies.

- *CORBA Interface Layer*: To support compiled applications (like Visual Basic or C++), a CORBA interface layer has been added to the above services. This layer provides protocol translation only. The request is then delegated to the EJB service layer.

- *Big Brother Monitoring*: Added test and reporting functionality to integrate with a public domain monitoring service, Big Brother.

Legacy Systems Integration

Vendor "best of class" transaction processing systems continue to operate as components within Vanderbilt's information architecture. However, such legacy systems are acquired and used in the context of the overall architectural philosophy, not just to address a specific task. For example, a vendor system that is otherwise "best of class" will not be purchased if it is unable to interface with other important aspects of the overall architecture. Major vendor systems include the following:

- McKesson HealthQuest Patient Management for inpatient ADT, outpatient surgery ADT, emergency department (ED) registration; HealthQuest Patient Accounting for technical billing; and HealthQuest Medical Records for case abstract and chart tracking;

- Epic Cadence and Resolute for outpatient clinic scheduling, registration, and professional billing;

- TripleG for clinical labs, microbiology, and anatomic pathology;

- Hemocare for blood bank;

- IDXRad for the radiology information system;

- AGFA for the radiology PACS;
- McKesson Series system for inpatient pharmacy;
- IPATH ORMIS for operative services; and
- Eclypsis for management decision support.

The use of these transaction processing systems is restricted to workflow within an operational area such as the laboratory. Data of interest to clinicians, educators, or administrators outside of an operational area are externalized to the repositories where the data can be accessed by appropriate tools that integrate into other workflows. Although it is increasingly possible for such applications and tools to share directly a single data repository, it is useful to treat the application database and the external database repository as distinct architectural layers to isolate corruption and to separate management of data that are work in progress from data that are in publishable form.

For example, laboratory test orders generated by WizOrder are printed on the patient's ward (as a part of the "requisition generation" process) with a bar-coded patient and test identifier, used for sample collection on the ward. At the same time that WizOrder generates the order, an electronic copy is sent via the GIE into an enterprise repository. Specimens arriving in the laboratory system are processed via LabTalk2, a middleware application that reads the bar code on the requisition, obtains the corresponding detailed order information via the GIE from the enterprise repository, passes required test-related and patient-related information into the laboratory system (via the GIE), and returns (via the GIE) an "in lab" status to update the repository. As results are generated in the laboratory system, they are handed to the GIE for transmission to StarChart for result reporting and escalation. Because all tests that are ordered do not result in specimens delivered to the laboratory, the foregoing system eliminates the need for a complex interface queue management between the order capture system and the laboratory system. It also provides a status tracking mechanism for all stages of laboratory test processing, from ordering, to performance, to resulting. Since integration is provided by the enterprise-wide ordering and repository layers, the laboratory has the freedom of using multiple simple systems that rely on the enterprise architecture, rather than requiring a large, complex, vertically integrated, and expensive laboratory information system.

Application Component Architecture

VUMC has adopted application component architecture standards for internal development of enterprise services and purchased software where practical.

The simplest user interface is used that meets the application requirements, starting with static HTML pages created off-line, progressing to server generated pages, then to pages that include Java applets, then to pages with compiled ActiveX components, and finally to a locally installed Java, C++, or Visual Basic (VB) client application.

The preferred framework for development of rules is EJB running under BEA WebLogic. CORBA Object Management Group (OMG) may be used as an alternative to the native EJB client access protocol.

Transactions that update the data repositories are routed through one of the communication engines described above, coupled with a transaction-processing monitor when practical. Reads of the data repositories are often direct from the database for performance reasons.

Oracle and DB2 are the enterprise structured data stores. Use of triggers and stored procedures is discouraged. Use of Java-coded stored procedures is the preferred compromise since the actual Java procedures can be moved to the middle tier as a migration path if the database management system changes.

Decision support is provided by a set of interrelated tools from four functional areas: data storage, metadata, reporting, and access. Data extracted from departmental financial, clinical, and research systems and stored in an Oracle enterprise data warehouse. Higher level data are aggregated and served to users by an array of Microsoft based datamarts. The array of datamarts on smaller servers allows scalable reporting for departments while maintaining high performance for real-time analysis. Data about the contents of the warehouse, the datamarts, and current reports are stored and Web accessed from a metadata repository, which was created using Lotus Notes. This is used by both technical staff as well as end-users to see what data elements, transformations, and reports exist. Tiered levels of reporting and analysis are provided. Static reports can be in any format, and currently include reports generated from Crystal Reports, Microsoft Excel, Business Objects, TRMS, and Adobe PDFs. Sets of logically linked Web-based executive reports are published using ProClarity. Web-based ad hoc reporting is done using Business Objects. On-line analytical processing (OLAP), with data cubes, uses a combination of Microsoft OLAP Services and ProClarity clients. All reports and metadata are accessed through a Web-based information portal, which also hosts departmental documents such as calendars of events, standard procedures, notices, etc. This portal was constructed using Lotus Notes, but is accessed using any Web browser.

Results

The information management infrastructure developed at Vanderbilt is in use throughout VUH and TVC. Indicators of its penetration include the following:

- Shared registration data across all inpatient and outpatient areas.
- Shared electronic patient chart across all inpatient and outpatient areas contains about 150 document types, and is used interactively 9,000 times per day by 2,200 distinct users.

- All inpatient units except the neonatal ICU and the Clinical Research Unit utilize WizOrder for all categories of orders, generating 7000 to 10,000 orders per day, on average 70% directly by physicians.
- 50% of inpatient units utilize PathworX.
- There are over 20,000 reports on the portal, and over 2,000 new reports are automatically generated quarterly.

Indications of the architecture's acceptance by the institution are reflected by two recent decisions:

- to complete the conversion to filmless radiology by the end of 2002; and
- to take the remaining paper-based processes out of the clinic by the end of 2002.

However, the change in organizational culture that it is nurturing is a more important indicator of its effectiveness. Access to data about VUMC practice patterns is being used to bring home to both clinical leadership and to individual physicians the fact that practice variability is a major fixable problem. For the first time, the organization has the will to systematically introduce evidence into practice. The Pharmacy and Therapeutics Committee is going beyond limiting the formulary, to recommending situations where drugs should be substituted because of increased efficacy and decreased cost. The Care Improvement Committee is developing complex treatment advisors for interventions such as the initiation of anticoagulation. The Resource Utilization Committee is specifying which imaging procedure is appropriate in a particular clinical situation. As knowledge such as these practices is developed throughout the organization, it is represented in the generalized external tables, and then linked into workflow by the appropriate tool to make it available when it can have an effect. The resulting change is tracked as a by-product of use of the tool, leading to refinement if needed.

Discussion and Conclusions

Based on the experience at VUMC with an *enterprise information architecture* (EIA), the following principles may generalize to other sites:

- Externalize data and business logic from "legacy" systems in application-independent repositories. A "legacy" system is one where meaning is implicit in code or process, or where data retrieval and storage are restricted within the system. The content of the repositories should be self-explanatory.
- Adopt industry standards where they exist, such as the HL7 messaging standard. If an existing resource is the best surrogate for a standard (such as SNOMED for clinical concepts), extend it. Where a resource is grossly inadequate (such as ICD for medical problems), map to it.

- If there are multiple sources for an item, represent both versions. An item has multiple sources if it is acquired through different processes with variation in meaning or accuracy.
- View individual systems as components (transaction processors, data capture devices, etc.), not as data repositories.
- Centralize global functions (ordering, notification, etc.) that can scale up and provide consistency across the enterprise. Role-specific user interfaces can shield users from the multitude of transaction processors needed to carry out their decisions.
- Use interface engine technology, augmented to support logical unit of work among distributed components, to mediate and to avoid a direct interface for each combination of participating systems.
- Support for evolutionary development and adaptation is more important than getting it right.

Acknowledgments

This work was supported in part by National Library of Medicine grant, Fast Track Provision of IAIMS, GO8-LM05443, National Institutes of Health, Department of Health and Human Services.

References

[Geissbuhler 1996] Geissbuhler A, Miller RA. A new approach to the implementation of direct care-provider order entry. *Proc AMIA Annu Fall Symp.* 1996; 689–693.

[Giuse 1996] Giuse DA, Mickish A. Increasing the availability of the computerized patient record. *Proc AMIA Annu Fall Symp.* 1996; 633–637.

[Ozbolt 1996] Ozbolt, J, Brennan G, Hatcher I. PathworX: an informatics tool for quality improvement. *Proc AMIA Symp* 2001; 518–522.

[Stead 1991a] Stead WW. Systems for the year 2000: the case for an integrated database. *MD Comput.* 1991; 8(2): 103–110.

[Stead 1991b] Stead WW, Borden RB, Boyarsky MW, Crow DS, Mears TP, Stone AA, Woods PJ. A system's architecture which dissociates management of shared data and end-user function. *Proc Annu Symp Comput Appl Med Care.* 1991; 475–480.

[Stead 1996] Stead WW, Borden R, Bourne J, Giuse D, Giuse N, Harris TR, Miller RA, Olsen AJ. The Vanderbilt University fast track to IAIMS: transition from planning to implementation. *JAMIA.* 1996; 3(5): 308–317.

Postface

I love and admire the past,
but I would like the future
to be even better.
—Romain Rolland

Managing Complexity

Hospital information systems grow not only by themselves but also through the development of organizational and technological networks. On the one hand, hospitals merge to improve their efficiency. They need to be linked with other institutions, insurance companies, governmental organizations, and general practitioners over wide area networks transporting sensitive patient information.

From the *user side*, data and services must be available anytime, anywhere, to anybody, eventually through the Internet, without endangering the integrity and security of the critical medical processes and patient information.

From the *human resource side*, as compared to other industries, hospitals are highly vulnerable since they must manage with a limited pool of computer specialists, and survive if the competition steals their best developers overnight. A turnover of computer staff always results in loss of continuity as departing staff members take with them hard-won knowledge gained over years.

From the *technology side*, important advances in computer-based technologies have taken place: a dramatic increase in computing power, combined with considerable advances in telecommunications systems and broadband networks. This rate of change in computer technology increases the risk that projects with a long project life cycle cause early technology choices to become obsolete even before the results of the project can be deployed.

Challenge of Software Engineering

While we are still witnessing the so-called software crisis, the software industry constantly rethinks how software needs to be developed with better efficiency and security. The key considerations are the ability to

- thoroughly understand the business domain and design systems that accurately model larger and larger parts of the perceivable reality,
- maintain the integrity of the system as the business domain evolves, and
- reduce the maintenance backlog and security trade-offs.

For more than two decades, the challenge of the software industry has been to achieve "software reusability" where standard components, selected from vendor catalogues, are customized to the specific needs of the client. However, the majority of reuse initiatives did not succeed as the culture of reuse was undervalued and tools were lagging behind.

Success in enterprise application development in the Internet age requires that information technology evolution must parallel business changes, and corresponding shifts in the way information technology managers face developments must be made. In this book we have described a strategy in which software design must be driven by a component-based approach. Applications are designed as collections of collaborating components that provide the conceptual metaphor necessary for the assembly of systems from a variety of sources that exist within a defined environment or component model. Application servers essentially provide the integration infrastructure in which components can be executed.

The list of components and the inner organization is neither exhaustive nor definitive. Names and functions of the components have been inspired in this book by the Healthcare Information System Architecture (HISA) propositions from the CEN/TC 251 standardization initiative (Comite Europeen de Normalisation–Technical Commitee 251 for medical Informatics. [www.centc251.org]). When it comes to actual implementation, components may largely vary in number and functional coverage. They are unlikely to be too numerous since the complexity of the overall system exponentially increases with their number.

Experience from Case Studies

Many software packages are considered monolithic, and they do not easily meet the needs of organizations or integrate with existing legacy applications for maximum operational efficiency within the organizational context. Two university hospitals (AZ-VUB in Brussels, HCUG in Geneva) have therefore decided to develop their own component-based solutions that are described in the case studies in this book. The HEGP in Paris and the VUMC in Nashville, in contrast, presents a best-of-breed approach on top of an integration middleware. All experiences emphasize the need for a sound enterprise integration architecture (EIA).

Although the cost of purchasing a package is less than the estimated cost of developing an application, there are often significant hidden costs related to customization and integration of commercial off-the-shelf (COTS) components. Some reports indicate that the cost of customization may rise to over 80% of the total cost of a package replacement project.

When moving from a traditional to a component-based approach several difficulties must be anticipated and recognized. Complexity increases when compared with traditional vertical solutions. A problem might arise from a single component, from the connection between two components, or from more complex relationships among components. Intervention in one area may have impacts that are difficult to anticipate and that eventually decrease the end-user confidence in the overall environment.

Many companies move and change; their requirements are rarely downsized, and they do not expect to lose systems management features in the process. In fact developments and implementation projects of component-based solutions are still complicated by the lack of system management tools as compared with the traditional client/server world.

Organizational and Human Aspects

This book focused on the technologic aspects of a component-based approach to the development of clinical information systems. This does not mean that the organizational or human aspect are not relevant or that technology solves these issues. Whatever the technology used, high participation from the end-user is unlikely to be achieved without a strong commitment by the decision makers and key leaders of the organization and the participation of representative users at every major decision step. For most end-users, clinical information systems will always remain "black boxes" managed by obscure computer scientists looking for the next generation software paradigm.

Glossary

access control. The management of permissions for logging on a computer system or network.

access control policy. A set of defined rules as part of a security policy, by which users are authenticated, granted, or denied access to applications and other services.

admission-discharge-transfer (ADT). Subsystem of a hospital information system that provides the function of patient admission, discharge, and transfer, and maintains the hospital census.

agent. Program that acts independently and intelligently (intelligent agent) to carry out a precise action. Agents are used on the World Wide Web to find information or to automatically index information.

ANSI. (American National Standards Institute). Organization that develops industrial standards, in particular recommendations for languages, electronic data exchange (EDI) and peripheral devices.

API. (application program interface). Software that provides a set of functions and resources to provide easy access to an application program.

applet. Small application that performs a specific task. JAVA applets make Web pages more interactive and dynamic.

application component. Units of application software that can be combined to produce larger units of functionality.

Application Server Page (ASP). A Web server technology from Microsoft that facilitates the creation of dynamic and interactive sessions with the user.

application service provider (ASP). An organization that provides users with application software via the Internet. Users pay for the software on the basis of their usage rather than purchasing a software licence.

Arden syntax. A computer language that provides means for writing medical rules relating patients and situations to actions to follow. Each module is called a medical logic module (MLM), which is made up of slots grouped into maintenance, library, and knowledge categories.

artificial intelligence (AI). The discipline concerned with building computer systems that perform functions that would be said to require intelligence if performed by humans or animals (or functions that might
otherwise be described as intelligent). AI is an interdisciplinary area with
inputs from computer science, psychology, neuroscience, cybernetics, lin-
guistics, and philosophy. AI is concerned with natural language understanding, machine learning, computer vision, machine reasoning, and
expert systems.

asymmetric encryption. Encoded information that can only be decoded
with a private key, usually a guarded password.

authentication. A process for positive and unique identification of users,
implemented to control system access.

authorization. The granting of rights, which includes the granting of access
based on access rights.

B2B. Business-to-business commerce via the Internet, for example, a hospital purchasing its supplies over the Internet.

B2C. Business-to-consumer commerce via the Internet, for example, an on-
line drugstore.

Backbone network. A high-speed communication network that carries
major traffic between smaller networks.

baud. Number of times per second that a carrier signal changes its state. In
practice, a 9600-baud modem transmits approximately 960 characters or
symbols per second. Only at very low rates is baud equal to bits per second
(bps).

biosignal processing. The monitoring of physiologic variables such as blood
pressure, heart rate, and temperature using instrumentation.

BPML. (Business Process Modeling Language). A metalanguage for the
modeling of business processes.

broadband. (1) High-speed transmission. (2) A method of transmitting data,
voice, and video using frequency division multiplexing, such as used with
cable TV.

bus. Set of conductors that transfer information between different parts of a
computer.

business object. A broad category of business processes that are modeled as
objects. A software construct that encapsulates description and behavior.
A business object can be as large as an order entry or a medical record system.

business component. The software implementation of an autonomous business concept or business process.

care activity. Activity which intends to improve or increase knowledge of the conditions of a subject of care.

CASE. (computer-aided software engineering). Environment to assist in software development.

case mix. Composition of cases in a group for a clinical trial such that no unwanted bias occurs.

case-based reasoning. A process in which a physician will check an earlier case at a diagnosis for a new patient.

CEN. (Comité Européen de Normalisation). European organization responsible for defining standards. Committee 251 (CEN TC251) is responsible for developing standards for information technology applied to health.

census. Statistic of bed usage in a hospital at a given time.

classification. Classification is the systematic placement of things or concepts into categories that share some common attributes or properties. A classification structure is a listing of terms that depicts hierarchical structures.

Clinical data repository (CDR). Clinical database optimized for storage and retrieval for information on individual patients and used to support patient care and daily operations.

clinical decision support system. Computer system designed to help health professionals make clinical decisions.

clinical information. Information about a patient, relevant to the health or treatment of that patient, that is recorded by or on behalf of a healthcare professional.

clinical information system (CIS). Information system that manages clinical data to support patient care and clinical decision making derived from various feeder systems such as laboratory, radiology, etc.

clinical investigation. Healthcare examination (laboratory, radiologic, or other) that leads to the production of one or more results.

clinical observation. Clinical information other than information about treatments and interventions.

clinical pathway. Disease-specific plan that identifies clinical goals, interventions, and expected outcomes by time period.

clinical protocol. A set of rules defining a standardized treatment program.

code value. The result of applying a coding scheme to a code meaning. Example: "CHF" as the representation of "congestive heart failure."

coded set. A set of elements that is mapped onto another set according to a coding scheme.

coding. The activity of using a coding scheme to map from one set of elements to another one.

coding scheme. A collection of rules that maps the elements of one set onto the elements of a second one.

common gateway interface (CGI). A small program that functions as a glue between HTML pages and other programs on a Web server.

community health information network (CHIN). A medical network that shares information.

compiler. A program that translates programs written in an advanced language (such as C, C++, or FORTRAN) into code executable by a computer. Compiled programs execute faster than interpreted programs.

component-based development (CBD). A software development approach where all aspects and phases of the development lifecycle are based on components.

computer-assisted diagnosis. Use of information technology for assisting healthcare professionals in diagnosis.

computer-assisted instruction (CAI). The application of computer technology to education. Also called computer-based training (CBT).

computer-assisted therapy. The application of computer technology to therapy.

computer-based patient record (CPR). See electronic patient record.

conformance testing. The testing of devices claimed to conform to certain standards to establish whether they actually do so.

consultation system. A teleradiology network used to discuss the findings of an examination with other physicians.

contrast resolution. The ability to distinguish between shades of gray on an image (see also spatial resolution).

CORBA. (Common Object Request Broker Architecture). An Object Management Group (OMG) standard that provides the standard interface definition between OMG-compliant objects.

critiquing system. Computer-based system that evaluates and suggests modifications for plans or data analyses already realized by a user.

cryptography. The conversion of data into a secret code for transmission over a public network. This discipline embodies principles, means, and methods for the transformation of data in order to hide their information content, prevent, undetected modification, and/or prevent their unauthorized use.

data compression. A technique that reduces the number of bits required to store data. Some compression techniques are designed to lose as little information as possible.

data confidentiality. Feature of an information system whereby data are made available to authorized entities only.

data integrity. Feature of an information system whereby information is protected from accidental or malicious alteration.

data item. Single unit of data that in a certain context is considered indivisible.

data security. Encompasses data confidentiality and availability.

DCOM. (Distributed Component Object Model). Microsoft's technology for distributed objects. Formerly Network OLE.

departmental system. System that supports a specific departmental functional activity within a healthcare environment, but that could also work as a stand-alone unit.

DES, 3DES. (Data Encryption Standard, Triple DES). A National Institute of Standards and Technology (NIST) standard for encrypting and decrypting data. A DES key has a 64-bit value; 8 bits are used to check parity, 56 bits for the encryption algorithm. Triple DES uses three 56-bit keys, for a total of 168 bits.

diagnosis related group (DRG). Group of patients defined using a case-mix approach based on homogeneous costs using major diagnosis, length of stay, secondary diagnosis, surgical procedure, age, and type of services required.

DICOM. (Digital Imaging and COmmunications in Medicine). A standard created by the American College of Radiology and the National Electrical Manufacturers Association to allow for the interchange of medical images and related information between computers and healthcare equipment produced by different manufacturers.

dictionary. Structured collection of lexical units containing linguistic information.

differential diagnosis. The set of active hypotheses (possible diagnoses) that a physician develops when determining the source of a patient's problem.

Diffie-Hellman. A cryptographic protocol that enables two parties to exchange public keys.

digital certificate. A digital equivalent of an identification card that is used in conjunction with a public key encryption system.

digital radiography. Computerized production, manipulation, and storage of radiographic images in digital format.

digital signature. Data appended to, or a cryptographic transformation of, a data unit that allows a recipient of a dat unit to prove the source and integrity of the unit.

distributed component (DC). A design pattern for an autonomous software artifact that can be deployed as a pluggable binary component into a run-time component execution environment.

DNS. (Domain Name System). Name resolution software to locate computers on a Unix or TCP/IP network.

domain name. The unique name that identifies an Internet site.

DSL. (Digital Subscriber Line). High-speed Internet access provided via a phone line.

e-commerce. Business transactions conducted over the Internet.

EDI. (electronic data interchange). The electronic communication of (business) transactions over a network.

EDIFACT. (Electronic Data Interchange For Administration Commerce and Transport). An ISO standard for electronic data interchange.

e-health. The market, companies, and initiatives for conducting health transactions over the Internet.

EJB. (Enterprise JavaBeans). A component software architecture from SUN Microsystems, used as the backbone of SUN's J2EE platform.

electronic health record (EHR). Collection of all the health related information about individual's life time stored in electronic format.

electronic patient record (EPR). Healthcare record stored in electronic format.

enterprise resource planning (ERP). An integrated information system that serves all departments within an enterprise.

firewall. Security software that prevents unauthorized access to a company's information technology (IT) infrastructure. The filtering performed by the firewall can occur at one or more levels of the network protocols.

flowsheet. A tabular summary of (medical) information that is arranged to display the values of variables as they change over time.

frame grabber. A device that captures a single still image from a video.

free-form text. Unstructured, uncoded representation of information in text format, for example, sentences describing the results of a patient's physical examination.

general message description (GMD). Subset of a domain information model prescribing the information content and semantic structure of a message.

GIF. (Graphics Interchange Format). Graphics format used for bitmap images. Often used on the WWW.

healthcare agent. Healthcare person, organization, device or software component that performs a role in a healtcare activity.

healthcare party. Organization or person involved in the direct or indirect provision of healthcare services to an individual or to a population.

health record entry. Data set, suitably attributed, which forms partof, or a whole, contribution to a health record at one place and time.

HELP. (Health Evaluation through Logical Process). The information and decision support system developed at LDS Hospital in Salt Lake City, Utah. It is the largest clinical decision support system in routine use. HELP provides decision support for many aspects of hospital practice, and can be considered a general hospital information system. HELP has a detailed nomenclature of findings, diseases, and procedures.

HISA. (Healthcare Information System Architecture). European Prestandard (prENV 12967, March 1997) proposed by CEN (Comité Européen de Normalisation) for the architecture of healthcare information systems.

HL7. (Health Level 7). A group created to develop standards to allow the interchange of healthcare-related textual data between computers and health care equipment produced by different manufacturers.

hospital information system (HIS). Generic term to describe one or more computer systems in a hospital designed to support the administrative and clinical services within the hospital.

HTML. (HyperText Markup Language). Page description language used on the Web.

HTTP. (HyperText Transfer Protocol). A communication protocol used to connect to servers on the Internet.

IAIMS. (Integrated Advanced Information Management Systems). An institution-wide computer network that links library systems with individual databases and information files within the institution's system or from outside the system for patient care, research, education, or administration.

image enhancement. Computer techniques used to improve the quality of an image (e.g., noise filtering, contrast sharpening).

image manipulation. Image processing function that does not change the contents of the image (e.g., translation, enlargement, rotation, and windowing).

image prefetching. A PACS system is based on a multiple-layer storage structure that contains all the images. Response times can be improved when images are prefetched from the low-level archive (optical, tape archive) to the high-level local buffer before they are requested.

image segmentation. The extraction of selected regions of interest from an image using automated or manual techniques.

imaging modality. A method for producing images (e.g., x-ray imaging, computed tomography, echosonography, and magnetic resonance imaging).

interchange format. Specification of a message type according to a given message syntax, covering the identification of the message type elements, their arrangements, representation and interrelationships.

Internet. Worldwide network of interconnected computers. Uses the TCP/IP communications protocol.

interpreter. Program that simultaneously translates and executes a program written in an advanced programming language (e.g., BASIC, LISP).

intranet. An inhouse Web site that serves the employees of the enterprise. A private network based on the Internet protocol.

IP. (Internet Protocol). The IP part of the TCP/IP communications protocol.

IP address. (Internet Protocol address). The unique address of a computer attached to a TCP/IP network Addresses are expressed as four sets of numbers separated by periods (e.g., 165.113.245.2).

IPsec. (IP Security). A widely used collection of security protocols developed and supported by the IETF (Internet Engineering Task Force), which allows for private and secure communications across the Internet.

ISDN. (Integrated Services Digital Network). Digital networking standard for high-speed transmission of data (documents, images, sound) over specialized telephone lines.

ISO. (International Organization for Standardization). An organization, founded in 1946, that sets international standards.

Java. An interpreted, object-oriented programming language developed by Sun Microsystems. Derived from C++, it lets programmers write interactive pieces of code, called *applets*, that may be downloaded from the Web at the same time as HTML pages.

JPEG. (Joint Photographic Experts Group). Image compression technique. The amount of information lost depends on the level of compression.

L2TP. (Layer 2 Tunneling Protocol). A merging of features from PPTP and Cisco's L2F. It is used to encapsulate PPP frames and transmit them across a TCP/IP network. As an IETF standard, L2TP is supported by many VPN providers.

JSP. (JavaServer Page). An extension to the Java servlet technology from SUN Microsystems. A JSP is an HTML page with embedded Java code that can call Enterprise JavaBeans (EJBs) for additional processing. An alternative

leased line. A private communications channel leased from a common carrier.

LDAP. (Lightweight Directory Access Protocol). Set of protocols for accessing information directories. Based on the X.500 standard, it is significantly simpler and supports TCP/IP.

legacy application. An application that has been in existence for some time (e.g., a mainframe application).

Linux. (Linus Unix). An implementation of the Unix kernel originally written from scratch with no proprietary code.

lossless compression. A compression technique that reduces the number of bytes to store data without losing information.

lossy compression. A compression technique that reduces the number of bytes to store data with loss of information.

master patient index (MPI). The module of a healthcare information system used to uniquely identify a patient.

M. Formerly known as MUMPS (Massachusetts General Hospital Utility Multi-Programming System). A programming language associated with an operating and database management system specially used in medicine.

MeSH. (Medical Subjects Heading). A thesaurus of over 18,000 medical terms used for the indexing of biomedical literature. MeSH consists of a set of headings arranged in a multilevel hierarchy. There are over 18,000 main headings in the primary structure of MeSH. The chemical supplement to MeSH contains about 50,000 chemical terms.

Medline. (MEDlars onLINE). An on-line bibliographic database of medical information provided by the National Library of Medicine (NLM).

MIB. (Medical Information Bus). IEEE P1073 standard proposed for data acquisition from a variety of medical devices.

MIME. (Multipurpose Internet Mail Extensions). The standard for attaching nontext files to standard Internet mail messages. Nontext files include graphics, spreadsheets, formatted word-processor documents, sound files, etc.

MPEG.. Motion Picture Experts Group). Video image compression format. Does not store each image, only the changes from one image to the next. One minute of animation requires approximately 9 MB of disk space.

multimedia record. Record that contains textual information and multimedia information (video, sound, animation, images, etc.).

narrowband. A telecommunications medium that uses low-frequency signals (50 bps–64 Kbps). Contrast with broadband.

natural language processing (NLP). The use of computers to interpret the meaning of natural language.

object. A functional entity that has a state and a defined set of operations. Objects can interact with one another. Any part of the perceivable or conceivable world.

object class. A set of objects possessing the same logical and functional properties.

order entry system. System for recording and processing orders.

outpatient. Patient who does not reside in a healthcare facility.

PACS. (Picture Archiving and Communication System).   System that can store, distribute, retrieve, and display images and related data.

patient card. Computer readable card held by or related to a patient.

pattern recognition. An automatic or semiautomatic process to recognize meaningful motifs.

PDA. (personal digital assistant). Handheld computer that serves as an organizer for personal information. Users can synchronize their PDAs with a PC or information system using a cradle device or a wireless communication system (infrared or radio-wave transmission, beaming).

pixel. (picture element). The smallest element or dot of a display. Image resolution improves as the number of pixels used by a display monitor increases.

plug-in. Auxiliary program that works with a major software program to enhance its capability.

point-of-care system. Information system that includes bedside workstations or other devices for capturing and entering data at the locations of patients.

portal. A Web site that provides a broad array of services and content.

PPP. (Point-to-Point Protocol). A TCP/IP-based protocol used to transmit IP packets over serial point-to-point links.

PPTP. (Point-to-Point Tunneling Protocol). A tunneling protocol developed by Ascend Communications, ECI Telecom, Microsoft, and U.S. Robotics that encapsulates PPP frames over TCP/IP networks. There is no standard implementation of PPTP.

privacy. The right of individuals to control or influence what information related to them may be collected and stored and by whom and to whom that information may be disclosed.

public key. The published part of a public key cryptography system. The private part is known only from the owner.

QMR. (Quick Medical Reference).   A decision support system developed from the Internist-1 expert system at University of Pittsburgh.

RSA. (Rivest–Shamir–Adleman). The public-key cryptographic system developed in 1977 by Ron Rivest, Adi Shamir, and Leonard Adleman. RSA is the most commonly used public-key encryption and authentication algorithm.

scanner. A device that creates a digital image either directly or by reconstructing a nondigital image.

semantic network. A formalism (often expressed graphically) for representing relational information, the arcs of the network representing the relationships and the nodes the objects in the network.

servlet. A Java program that extends the functionality of a Web server, generating dynamic content and interacting with Web clients using a request-response paradigm.

SGML. (Standard Generalized Markup Language). An ISO formal description language for hypertext documents.

SNOMED. (Systematized Nomenclature of Medicine). A multiaxial nomenclature for the coding of medical and health-related terms.

spatial resolution. The ability to distinguish between adjacent structures an an image. See also contrast resolution.

SQL. (Structured Query Language). Language used to interrogate relational databases. This is a fourth-generation language.

static image. An image with characteristics that do not change. Such an image requires less electronic storage space and bandwidth than a video.

store-and-forward technology. The process in which data can be stored and transmitted electronically at a later time, rather than immediately during the acquisition process.

subject of care. Person scheduled to receive, receiving, or having received healthcare.

T1. A 1.544 Mbps high-speed point-to-point connection on lines leased by telephone companies.

T3. A 44.736 Mbps high-speed point-to-point connection on lines leased by telephone companies.

TCP/IP. (Transmission Control Protocol/ Internet Protocol). Set of communications standards (protocols) for transferring data (and for error correction) from one computer to another over the Internet.

telemedicine. The delivery of health care at distance (e.g., via the Internet or telecommunication tools).

teleradiology. The remote interpretation of medical images.

Telnet. A terminal emulation protocol commonly used on TCP/IP-based networks and the Internet.

thesaurus. A comprehensive list of subjects concerning which information may be retrieved by using the proper key terms.

UDDI. (Universal Description, Discovery, and Integration). An XML-based specification for worldwide registry of Web services for publishing, discovery, and integration purposes.

UML. (Unified Modeling Language). A standardized object-oriented analysis and design language from the Object Management Group (OMG).

UMLS. (Unified Medical Language System). A large terminology project developed under the direction of the National Library of Medicine (NLM) to produce a unified thesaurus and cross reference linking various medical nomenclatures. The UMLS includes an information sources directory, a metathesaurus, and a semantic net.

UNIX. Operating system developed by Bell Laboratories in the early 1970s, now widely used on minicomputers and workstations.

USB. (Universal Serial Bus). A hardware standardized interface for low-speed peripheral devices such as a keyboard or a mouse.

W3C. (World Wide Web Consortium). An international consortium founded in 1994 to develop standards for the World Wide Web.

WAIS. (Wide Area Information Server). UNIX server on the Internet that contains indexes to documents.

Web. Short for the World Wide Web. See WWW.

wireless LAN (WLAN). Local area network that uses radio frequency technology to transmit data for relatively short distances.

WWW. (World Wide Web). Hypertext system that links together documents over the Internet.

WYSIWYG. (What You See Is What You Get). Term used to describe graphics systems in which the information displayed on the screen is the same as what will be printed.

XML. (eXtensible Markup Language). A subset of the Standard Generalized Markup Language (SGML) that is designed to make it easy to interchange structured documents over the Internet. Controlled by the World Wide Web Consortium (W3C).

XSL. (eXtensible Stylesheet Language). A style sheet format for XML documents.

XSLT. (eXtensible Stylesheet Language Transformation). A language to covert an XML document into another XML, HTML, or other format document.

Index

Health Informatics Series
(formerly Computers in Health Care)

(continued from page ii)

Behavioral Healthcare Informatics
N.A. Dewan, N.M. Lorenzi, R.T. Riley, and S.R. Bhattacharya

Patient Care Information Systems
Successful Design and Implementation
E.L. Drazen, J.B. Metzger, J.L. Ritter, and M.K. Schneider

Introduction to Nursing Informatics, Second Edition
K.J. Hannah, M.J. Ball, and M.J.A. Edwards

Information Retrieval
A Health and Biomedical Perspective, Second Edition
W.R. Hersh

Information Technology for the Practicing Physician
J.M. Kiel

Computerizing Large Integrated Health Networks
The VA Success
R.M. Kolodner

Medical Data Management
A Practical Guide
F. Leiner, W. Gaus, R. Haux, and P. Knaup-Gregori

Organizational Aspects of Health Informatics
Managing Technological Change
N.M. Lorenzi and R.T. Riley

Transforming Health Care Through Information
Case Studies
N.M. Lorenzi, R.T. Riley, M.J. Ball, and J.V. Douglas

Trauma Informatics
K.I. Maull and J.S. Augenstein

Public Health Informatics and Information Systems
P.W. O'Carroll, W.A. Yasnoff, M.E. Ward, L.H. Ripp,
and E.L. Martin

Advancing Federal Sector Health Care
A Model for Technology Transfer
P. Ramsaroop, M.J. Ball, D. Beaulieu, and J.V. Douglas

Medical Informatics
Computer Applications in Health Care and Biomedicine, Second Edition
E.H. Shortliffe and L.E. Perreault

Filmless Radiology
E.L. Siegel and R.M. Kolodner

Cancer Informatics
Essential Technologies for Clinical Trials
J.S. Silva, M.J. Ball, C.G. Chute, J.V. Douglas, C.P. Langlotz, J.C. Niland,
and W.L. Scherlis

Clinical Information Systems
A Component-Based Approach
R. Van de Velde and P. Degoulet

Knowledge Coupling
New Premises and New Tools for Medical Care and Education
L.L. Weed